"Cole writes close to the heart in his personal story of living with Parkinson's disease. . . . For those beginning their own journey through illness, as well as those who can look back at earlier paths traveled, this volume is likely to provide easily accessible comfort, perspective, and hope for joy yet to be discovered and savored. Wise readers may find themselves returning to this book more than once."

—KAREN RAPHAEL
Professor, New York University, and person living with Parkinson's disease

"As a young-onset Parkinson's disease (YOPD) patient myself, I struggled in my early years living with this illness. . . . Cole's experiences can serve the YOPD community with great impact. He provides incredible insight and perspective as a husband, father, educator, and friend living with Parkinson's. He has also found a balance in bringing hope though honesty while not sugarcoating the challenges we all face in all aspects of our lives."

—JIMMY CHOI
Contestant, American Ninja Warrior, and Member, Patient Council, The Michael J. Fox Foundation for Parkinson's Research, and person living with Parkinson's disease

"As a 'PwP' (person with Parkinson's), I found *Discerning the Way* both inspiring and revelatory. Cole writes with precision, grace, and empathy. His meditations on Parkinson's . . . provide us with a road map for hope, a path from darkness into light. This is a remarkable book of deeply personal stories that open a wide window into living well with Parkinson's."

—ERIC EYRE
Author of *Death in Mud Lick: A Coal Country Fight against the Drug Companies That Delivered the Opioid Epidemic*, and person living with Parkinson's disease

"The knowledge spectrum for a Parkinson specialist and researcher . . . is a broad scope, but still interpreted and acted upon from the perspective of the physician, no matter how empathetic. This collection of insight, anecdote, and inspiration from an observer so uniquely positioned reminds the health care provider that a completely different perspective exists—that hope, honesty, relationships, and humor impact chronic illness as much as, or more than, medicines and surgeries."

—WILLIAM G. ONDO, MD
Director, Movement Disorders Clinic, Houston Methodist Neurological Institute

"Parkinson's is a complicated disease that affects patients, caregivers, and others deeply and in a variety of ways. Cole delves into the illness with an insightful eye, one particularly focused on the experiences of young-onset patients, to share life lessons and perspectives that go beyond Parkinson's and apply to everyone, whether they suffer from PD or another disease. Optimistic yet not sugarcoating things, Cole candidly shares incredible observations and revelations with clarity and compassion."

—BRET I. PARKER
Co-chair, Patient Council, The Michael J. Fox Foundation for Parkinson's Research,
and person living with Parkinson's disease

"Cole has made a major contribution to the body of Parkinson's literature. Cole's message is clear: life is worthwhile and there is strength 'in removing the freight of going it alone.' His powerful and deeply personal style of storytelling draws in the reader in each essay with charm, wit, and insightfulness. . . . This is an essential read for anyone with Parkinson's."

—NINA MOSIER, MD
Co-founder and Director, Power for Parkinson's

"This is a profoundly important book—deeply human, beautifully written, and at times even poetic. . . . Cole helps us understand the physiological and emotional daily challenges for people living with PD, at the same time as he outlines a pathway to hope and meaning. . . . This book will leave a lasting impact on readers, reminding us of our frailties and our strengths, our interdependence, and the empowering effect that comes from living authentically even when dealing with loss."

—JEANETTE R. DAVIDSON
Professor and former Director, The Clara Luper Department of African
and African American Studies, University of Oklahoma

"*Every word* of Cole's book resonates to the core with me, even though parts of my experience with PD are quite similar and parts are quite different. . . . I highly recommend this book for those with Parkinson's and their care partners, physicians, nurses, social workers—anyone, really, who cares to know more about what living, and thriving, with Parkinson's can look like."

—NICOLE JARVIS, MD, OB/GYN
Physician, and person living with Parkinson's disease

"Cole's beautifully written book is packed with wisdom, not only for those with chronic illness but for *all of us*. For me, this intimate account reads like a spiritual memoir—a profound and honest journey with human mortality in which Cole confronts and transforms an unexpected diagnosis into an occasion for learning. And we learn so much, not just about Parkinson's but about the practice of mercy, gratitude, and resilience amid life's many losses."

—BONNIE J. MILLER-MCLEMORE
E. Rhodes and Leona B. Carpenter Professor Emerita of Religion, Psychology, and
Culture, Vanderbilt University Divinity School

DISCERNING THE WAY

DISCERNING THE WAY

Lessons from Parkinson's Disease

Allan Hugh Cole, Jr.

CASCADE *Books* · Eugene, Oregon

DISCERNING THE WAY
Lessons from Parkinson's Disease

Cascade Books
An Imprint of Wipf and Stock Publishers
199 W. 8th Ave., Suite 3
Eugene, OR 97401

www.wipfandstock.com

PAPERBACK ISBN: 978-1-7252-9957-3
HARDCOVER ISBN: 978-1-7252-9958-0
EBOOK ISBN: 978-1-7252-9959-7

Cataloguing-in-Publication data:

Names: Cole, Allan Hugh, Jr., author.

Title: Discerning the way : lessons from Parkinson's disease / Allan Hugh Cole, Jr.

Description: Eugene, OR: Cascade Books, 2021 | Includes bibliographical references.

Identifiers: ISBN 978-1-7252-9957-3 (paperback) | ISBN 978-1-7252-9958-0 (hardcover) | ISBN 978-1-7252-9959-7 (ebook)

Subjects: LCSH: Cole, Allan Hugh, Jr. | Parkinson's disease—Patients—United States—Biography. | Life change events—Psychological aspects. | Meaning (Psychology).

Classification: RC382 .C55 2021 (paperback) | RC382 (ebook)

12/20/21

The author would like to express his gratitude to Oxford University Press for permission to use or adapt material from Allan Hugh Cole, Jr., *Counseling Persons with Parkinson's Disease,* Copyright © 2021 by Oxford University Press.

For Holly and Meredith, who help me discern the way.

"Do not spoil what you have by desiring what you have not; remember that what you now have was once among the things you only hoped for."

—Epicurus

"Don't tell me the moon is shining;
show me the glint of light on broken glass."

—Anton Chekhov

CONTENTS

PREFACE

On October 26, 2016, how I see the world changed, as did my imagined future. A neurologist I had only just met uttered these soul-shaking words: *What worries me is that I think you are in the early stages of Parkinson's disease.* I was forty-eight years old.

This book details the beginning of my journey with young-onset Parkinson's, a diagnosis given to those under the age of fifty. The four years since my diagnosis have been difficult at times, but also enlightening and redemptive. I will not realize my dream to pitch for the Houston Astros, but physical challenges, while bothersome, have not yet become limiting. Some things are harder to do, such as buttoning a shirt, getting a good night's sleep, and keeping symptoms at bay when under stress, and some days I feel more fatigued than I used to, but I can still do what I have always done. Of course, limitations will come at some point because this is how Parkinson's works.

Sadness, fear, worry, and uncertainty about the future have presented by far the greatest challenge. Early in my journey, the personal decline I imagined and dreaded, coupled with not wanting to burden my family, weighed on me. A lot. Dark thoughts left me anxious and without hope, and I assumed incorrectly that my best days were behind me. I have since discovered that others diagnosed with Parkinson's disease and with other progressive illnesses have similar thoughts and feelings.

With the support and encouragement of many people, including my family, friends, colleagues, and especially others who live with Parkinson's, I found ways to push through the darkness, and I eventually discovered a path forward and gained new insights that calmed my shaken soul. Chief among these insights is that although a serious illness presents profound challenges and losses, it can also lead to unanticipated gains. For me, these gains have included deeper and more authentic relationships; opportunities for reconciliation, personal growth, and gaining wisdom; profound gratitude, spiritual clarity, and newfound purpose, hope, and joy. In offering my insights on these gains—what I have come to call the *gifts* of Parkinson's—even as I still struggle sometimes, I hope to inspire others on a similar journey, especially those trying to find their own path forward.

I wrote part of my story to share because I am both a writer and a teacher. For nearly two decades, it has been my privilege, in the classroom and through writing, to teach others about subjects close to my heart. I taught counseling courses in a small seminary for eleven years, where most students go to learn how to be ministers and chaplains. Currently, I teach in a school of social work within a large public university. In both of these settings, writing and teaching have shaped my self-understanding, identity, and sense of purpose. These pursuits have also been sources of personal transformation and growth.

Much of this book appeared first on my blog, PD Wise (PDWise.com), which I launched in April of 2019. There, I write regularly about my experience with Parkinson's because it helps me find meaning and purpose in having this illness, and because writing about it helps me heal and live well, even as I face the uncertainty of life ahead. I also want to help others discover their own meaning, purpose, healing, and wellness, whether they live with Parkinson's disease or face other significant life challenges and uncertainties. In fact, while this book, like PD Wise, conveys my personal story with Parkinson's, it focuses as well on new opportunities and unexpected gains that can emerge from most any hardships, whatever their forms. My experience with Parkinson's provides a lens for bringing this broader focus into clearer view.

The essays in this book move back and forth in time and detail the *lessons* I am learning from Parkinson's. I do not have these lessons down pat, or learned once and for all. One cannot learn them by cramming, nor by parroting others, nor by rote memory. Rather, these lessons unfold each day, little by little, through living life, enduring its setbacks, recognizing its beauty, and nurturing oneself and others through love. A slow unfolding of these lessons comes with greater insight and clarity, but sometimes more confusion, too. Learning often happens this way. I am learning as I go, gradually becoming more aware, knowledgeable, and, I hope, wise, even as new questions arise, perplex me, and call for deeper exploration. There are additional lessons to learn, of course, but the ones described in this book seem like a good place to begin. As the ancient Greek philosopher Plato observed, "The beginning in every task is the chief thing."[1]

I also hope this book provides a personal testimony for my daughters, Meredith and Holly. Ages ten and eight when I was diagnosed, and now aged fifteen and thirteen, who they are and what they do provides me precious daily lessons in the virtues of hope, will, purpose, competence, fidelity, love, care, and wisdom.[2] Collectively, Mer and Holls are my heart and my soul, and my desire to remain an active part of their lives, to watch them grow up and thrive, and dance at their weddings sustains me. No doubt, they will need to write their own stories in the face of life's difficulties. As they do, may they know with certainty that their father, who loves them so deeply, finds peace, learns, grows, experiences new joys, teaches, writes, and lives well in the face of his own difficulties; and may they see that from personal hardships, whether our own or others', we can learn some of life's most important lessons.

Allan Cole
Austin, Texas
October 6, 2020

---

1. Plato, *The Republic*, Book I, 377-B.

2. These virtues are what psychologist Erik H. Erikson described as *strengths* that, when developed, help human beings thrive, psychologically, spiritually, and relationally.

ACKNOWLEDGMENTS

Wordsworth challenged writers to "Fill your paper with the breathings of your heart." This I have tried to do; and each of my heart's breathings has joined with deep gratitude for those who have inspired, encouraged, supported, and companioned me in my efforts to discern the way with Parkinson's disease.

Rodney Clapp, my wise and perceptive editor and a friend for many years, provided thoughtful guidance that helped me improve this book. The entire team at Cascade, which continues to set a high bar in publishing, also made significant contributions to this project. In particular, I want to thank Matthew Wimer, Managing Editor, and Ian Creeger, Lead Production Editor, for their assistance and good work. I am grateful to have worked with such stellar colleagues and persons.

Speaking of stellar persons, Elizabeth Gaucher, Principal at Longridge Editors and a dear friend for over thirty years, read most of this manuscript and provided keen insights and invaluable feedback that enriched the work, as did Ethan Henderson, my close friend and fellow young-onset Parkinson's journeyer. Both are smart and gifted writers and thinkers whose advice and friendship I benefit from and cherish.

I also owe a debt of gratitude to Jane von Mehren and Lauren Sharp, my agents at Aevitas Creative Management, whose patience, generosity, and constructive feedback has allowed me to grow as a writer.

A few chapters in this book, or portions of chapters, first appeared in another book I wrote just prior to this one, titled *Counseling Persons with Parkinson's Disease*. I am grateful to Oxford University Press for granting me permission to include this previously published work, and particularly for Dana Bliss, Executive Editor, for his generosity of friendship, support, and encouragement for writing and for living well with the Parkinson's beast.

When I think of friendship and support, several additional people who live with Parkinson's come to mind: Allison Toepperwein, Bret Parker, Bill Bucklew, Jimmy Choi, Chris Tracy, Jonathan Mackin, Chris Lion, Bob Sahm, Craig Potts, Kathy Holden, Ned Neuhaus, Dan Stultz, Joyce Chu, and Liz Miller, among many others. Several of these friends began their own journey with Parkinson's before I did and they welcomed me to this extraordinary community and this new life with kindness, compassion, and love. By virtue of their examples of courage and resolve to live a full life with this illness, they inspire me to do the same.

I am also grateful for my colleagues in the Steve Hicks School of Social Work at The University of Texas at Austin for helping me grow as a teacher, scholar, administrator, and person. A special word of gratitude extends to my team in the Office of Academic Affairs: Tanya Voss, Cossy Hough, Sarah Swords, Cynthia Franklin, Andrea Montgomery, Jennifer Luna, Ramón Gómez, Marian Mahaffey, Sherry Melecki, Eden Blesener, Jinane Sounny-Slitine, Alexis Kyle, Desiree Pacheco, Megan Randolph, Laura Dupuis, and Mia Vinton, my administrative assistant extraordinaire. All of these colleagues model the kind of work, service, and humanity of which we need more in the world.

Not long after I shared my diagnosis publicly, a friend introduced me to Nina Mosier and Susan Stahl, co-founders of Power for Parkinson's (PFP), a nonprofit organization that provides free exercise, singing, and dance classes to persons with Parkinson's (PwP) in the Austin area and around the world through online platforms. Soon thereafter, Nina and Susan invited me to join PFP's Board of Directors, work that has enriched my life by allowing me to become a part of a vibrant community and to connect with others seeking to live a full and meaningful life with Parkinson's. I am in their debt.

In a span of four years, a Parkinson's diagnosis has broken my heart and opened it, taxed my mind and freed it, and bound me to a new kind of life, one full of anticipated limitations *and* unanticipated meaning and joy. No greater meaning, nor joy, have I found than being Tracey's partner, Meredith and Holly's dad, Allan and Jeri's son, and sharing this Parkinson's journey with them. As the Psalmist declared, "the boundary lines have fallen for me in pleasant places" (Psalm 16:6a).

1

PARKINSON'S EYES

"The real voyage of discovery consists not in seeking new landscapes,
but in having new eyes."

—Marcel Proust

SEEING DIFFERENTLY

Having Parkinson's disease can affect your eyes. As a movement disorder, Parkinson's can make it harder to focus because it's more difficult to move your eyes quickly; and, because you don't blink as much, it can lead to excessively dry eyes as well, which causes discomfort and fatigue.

Since my Parkinson's diagnosis at the age of forty-eight, my eyes often get dry.

But I see things differently, too.

It's around 6 PM, and I am on my way home from The University of Texas at Austin campus. I decide to stop by my local Walgreens pharmacy to pick up a prescription for rasagiline, my daily Parkinson's medication. As I wait in line, a woman in front of me speaks with the pharmacy tech. I suppose that this woman is in her sixties. Overweight and using a cane, her bloated face, blotchy skin, and multiple sores on her hands and arms suggest years of poor health. A faded floral dress and frayed cloth handbag that rest on the pharmacy counter make me think she lives on meager resources, and the two-inch hole in the heel of her shoe tells a similar story.

I am not eavesdropping, but I hear part of her conversation with the pharmacy tech.

"I absolutely have to have *those* pills," she says, pointing to a small white bag in the tech's hand. "And I can wait on the others 'til next time," she says, pointing at two other white bags on the counter. "I'll get those when I get my check."

She has made these kinds of choices before.

I imagine that trying to decide which medicine to take, and which ones to wait on, feels like having to choose between food and water, or clothing and shelter. My stomach tightens up.

As the pharmacy tech gets the revised order ready, the woman steps away from the counter. She walks slowly to a nearby aisle to put other items that are in her shopping basket back on the shelf. She will have to wait to buy these, too.

One other person stands in line behind me. As I turn around, he sighs and shakes his head, and looks down at his Apple watch.

A different pharmacy tech calls me to the counter. I tell him my name, and he turns around and begins looking on a shelf for my single bag in the white plastic alphabetized bins. If I had no health insurance, my medicine would cost nearly $700 for a month's supply. That's the cost of a month's rent in many places. I prepare to give him my $10 co-pay. While I wait, I think about the woman waiting and of what she cannot afford.

It is as if I now possess laser eyes with a state-of-the-art guidance system for recognizing people facing adversity, hardships . . . pain.

I can easily pick out of the crowd the young man who walks to class with forearm crutches and metal leg braces, the same way I presume he has gotten around his entire life. I can hone in on the little girl at my kids' school, who pushes against her autism to join her classmates in the school program. I ache when I see my colleague whose husband has recently committed suicide, and when I think of the struggles that she and her eight-year-old daughter will face. And my thoughts linger on the parents of Harrison Brown, a University of Texas freshman. A student with severe mental illness killed him on campus in the spring of 2017, a few days before the end of the academic year. A few weeks later, Harrison's father, Kurt, succumbed to his own neurologic disease, amyotrophic lateral sclerosis (ALS), also known as Lou Gehrig's disease.

My Parkinson's eyes now lock on people living with illness, disability, poverty, discrimination, or hopelessness. I have been able to catch glimpses of these maladies before, for most of my life, in fact; but since my Parkinson's diagnosis, they pop with refractions I have never before imagined, much less seen.

SEEING OUR CONNECTEDNESS

For several months after my diagnosis, when I assumed my life was essentially over, I asked myself so many questions: How can I cope with having a progressive neurologic disease? With the challenges and complications that increase over time? With the unpredictability of any given day, much less a longer course of disease progression? How can I manage to live with these burdens?

I've learned that one way is by seeing personal struggles not as unique—which can lead to feelings of isolation and loneliness—but as part of a broader human landscape, where facing and coping with life's hardships will, eventually, be everyone's lot. All of us will face illness or other difficulties. This is just how life goes.

Understanding this facet of life, the philosopher Friedrich Nietzsche put it well: "To live is to suffer and to survive is to find meaning in the suffering."

Viewing Parkinson's in this fashion helps unite my own experiences of hardship with those of others, whether their burden is Parkinson's or something else, and this unity can prompt us, collectively, to see all who struggle with eyes of compassion, empathy, and respect. Still, seeing in this new way does more. Reminding us that we travel burdensome roads with others, and not alone, it births a conviction of solidarity, of togetherness. It's the conviction that, *together*, we can strive to ease our own plight *and* that of others; that, together, we can do something good with our infirmity; that, together, we can and will find new meanings, ones that help us not merely to survive but to flourish in whatever our new voyage of discovery becomes.

SEEING HOPE

One Sunday, my family and I are at the Austin Mennonite Church. Around noon, when the service has ended, a man about my age approaches me at the back of the sanctuary. Since he is wearing tattered and slightly dingy clothes, and has put several duffle bags in the corner of the room, I assume he lives on the street. Transient folks routinely visit this church, which embraces social, racial, and economic justice as part of its core mission. Everyone is welcome. No one gets turned away. Sometimes those who wander in want money or food. More often, they want human connection and reasons to hope.

After I introduce myself to this man, whose name is Joe, he holds out his arm, rolls up his sleeve, and shows me several painful looking sores. From his wrist past his elbow, his arm looks puffy and, in multiple places, oozes blood-tinged yellow pus.

"I'm afraid it's getting infected," he says. "I can't get up to the clinic 'til next week, but I reckon things'll work out."

I think of the story of Jesus and the beggar, Lazarus, who was covered with sores that were licked by dogs, and who longed to eat the crumbs that fell from the rich man's table.

We are having a potluck meal that day, so I invite Joe to make himself a plate of food. He does, and with it piled high, he takes a seat at the table. I wonder how often he gets to do that.

As I glance back at Joe, who is still enjoying his meal, I remember Kate, a middle-aged woman who also lives on the streets. She had wandered in to church on a different Sunday and I met her in front of the coffee pot. The clean white coffee cup stood in stark contrast to her dirty fingernails and the dinge of homelessness that covered her. She heard voices and seemed scared and suspicious.

As Joe continues to eat his lunch and talk with new friends, my daughter, Holly, and I walk across the street to the CVS drugstore and buy peroxide, antibiotic ointment, and bandages. When we return, Holly hands the paper bag to Joe. Looking inside, he tears up and puts his hand over his eyes. She looks at me and smiles, and then darts to the table of food to make herself a plate. She starts on the end with the desserts.

Joe lets his hand fall back to his side and looks at me, his eyes still moist and slightly red.

"Thank you, brother," he says. "I don't know what to say."

"You're welcome," I say, "and it's our pleasure."

We shake hands and Joe smiles before making another pass by the food table, putting some rolls in his pocket, and walking out of the church.

I hope he got to the clinic.

2

A MARATHON, NOT A SPRINT

At 4:45 AM on Sunday, eleven days after my Parkinson's diagnosis at the age of forty-eight, I awake to the sound of the door lock's firm click as my wife, Tracey, leaves our hotel room on Manhattan's Upper West Side. She and our close friend Stacey are catching the ferry to Staten Island together, where the New York City Marathon begins. We have decided to share the news of my diagnosis with Stacey and her husband, Paul, but no one else knows.

Our family had been excited about this trip for over a year, ever since Tracey decided to run the Marathon. She was an avid runner in college and when we first married, but gave it up for two decades before getting the running bug again. Once she did, she wanted to run her first marathon. Since she grew up on Long Island, it had to be New York.

As Meredith and Holly sleep, I lie in bed and listen to their gentle rhythmic breathing. Only a faint siren in the distance interrupts their sweet melodic sounds. I think of when they were little, and of the nights when they both wound up in our bed and I could smell lavender Aveeno baby shampoo on their hair. More than ever, the enormity of parenthood grips me.

Since it is still too early to get out of bed, I replay the previous few weeks, from the time I first noticed my finger tremor until I learned of my disease. A growing heaviness covers my chest as several toes on my left foot begin to cramp—something called *dystonia*. I have experienced it in both of my feet for a couple of years. Though a common Parkinson's symptom, I assumed I simply needed to eat more bananas.

Except for faint light peeking through the top of a closed curtain, darkness fills the room. Clouds of questions roll in, as they have every night since my visit with Dr. T, my neurologist and new best friend.

How will Tracey respond as I slow down and become less physically capable?

What if, down the road, I need help with everyday tasks?

Will her compassion turn into pity?

How long will I be able to work?

Will I be able to pay for my kids' college?

How will our plans for the future change?

. . . And how will our girls deal with all of this?

As my mind tries to field its own rapid-fire questions, it also scrolls through a range of scenarios. None can pierce the enveloping darkness.

***

Tracey and I were a few months shy of celebrating our twenty-fifth wedding anniversary when we learned I have Parkinson's. A social worker by training, she was employed in nursing homes and hospitals for the first thirteen years of our marriage, until we had Meredith. Geriatric social work suited her perfectly. Raised in the home of her grandparents, she had a love for older adults, and her disposition and personal strengths aligned perfectly with their needs. She is a born nurturer who has never met a stranger.

From the time she began this work, when we were in our early twenties, I often joked that she was my "long-term investment" and that I would have an "in" with a good nursing home when I needed one. Now in my late forties, and in what I had assumed was still the prime of life, I was not ready to begin drawing on this investment.

***

Later that morning, Meredith, Holly, and I, along with Tracey's cousins Tom and Peter, make our way from below the Atlantic Avenue subway station in Brooklyn up to the street. As we get to the top of the stairs, a majestic blue sky bursts over the city and a light, unseasonably warm breeze blows. It invites pleasant smells from a half-dozen street food vendors to collide, which my daughters notice with delight.

"Yuuuuum!" says Meredith, "love me some funnel cakes!"

"Oh yeah," Holly says, as she does a dance called "The Floss."

Meredith joins in.

"We'll get something after we see Mom. We don't want to miss her," I say, trying to keep us all on task.

As a band with four middle-aged men plays loud music on the large sidewalk, an AC/DC song, our pace quickens. We walk a couple of blocks, starting and stopping as we make our way through thick crowds. Holly, who is nine, holds my hand tightly. Meredith, who is eleven, has reached the age of rejecting my offers to hold hands, but she stays close, too, sandwiched between Tom and me. Searching for an opening along the route up 4th Avenue, I spot an area that will allow all of us to see the runners as they approach. People are friendly as we hurry to get there and snake our way through.

When we get to our waiting spot, I take in the scene. People smile and sway as another band plays nearby. Groups of runners pass steadily by. One spectator, a man wearing a white shirt with bright yellow smiley faces on it, holds a handmade sign. It reads, "Life is Good!" Staring at him fiercely, I almost flip him the bird and yell "Bullshit!"

My daughters' voices bring me back.

"Is she close, Daddy?" Holly asks.

"I hope she gets here soon, I'm hungry," Meredith says.

Meredith takes hold of the cowbell we have brought from Austin. Holly positions a sign they have made. It reads, *Go Mom . . . Bib #29292.*

After glaring back at the man holding the smiley face sign one more time, I pry my eyes away and look at the phone app that I am using to track Tracey's progress. I tell the girls when she gets to mile seven, and we begin scanning the colorful sea of runners in search of our pearl.

Each runner has a story, and I suppose each story has elements of both joy and sadness, calm and worry, hope and despair. This is the way life is.

I notice a few other signs in the crowd, including one that reads The Michael J. Fox Foundation for Parkinson's Research, and several groups of runners are wearing Team Fox jerseys.[1] Without thinking, I stick my fist in the air and yell, "Go Team Fox!" as one of the groups passes us. One of the runners looks over at me and pumps his fist in the air.

---

1. Part of the Michael J. Fox Foundation, which raises money for Parkinson's research, Team Fox members take part in various running, cycling, climbing, and other athletic events, including triathlons.

Never missing anything, Holly asks, "Who are you cheering for, Daddy?"

"For Team Fox, my love."

Meredith interjects, saving me from any further explanation or commentary.

"How much longer, Dad?"

"Very soon, Mer."

The first time we see her that warm autumn morning is at mile eight. Her purple New Balance shoes, which match the color of her headband and shirt, cushion her gazelle-like stride as she moves in cadence up 4th Avenue. The look of joy on her face makes me tingle. Seeing her outpace many younger men makes me smile. I wave both of my arms high in the air and yell, "Tray!" She sees me and runs toward us, flashing the same inviting smile—equal parts kind and comedic—that captured me a quarter of a century earlier in Boston. We all let out cheers and take turns hugging her. The girls hold onto their mom tightly.

"Get moving. You have eighteen miles to go!" I say.

She touches her hand quickly to her lips two times and extends it to meet mine. Our eyes lock.

"I love you, Allan," she says.

"I love you," I say, trying to slow my quivering lip. "Go run like the wind."

She smiles, blows me a kiss, and, always the zany soul, takes a few strides before turning around and running backwards. She adds several half bows (technically, she does a dance called the Dab).

I give her a thumbs up. She smiles, turns, and is absorbed back into the colorful sea.

I smile back at her. My sunglasses hide my red, moist eyes.

We see her two more times, at mile nineteen and again just before she crosses the finish line in Central Park. It is now cooler and cloudy. Her pace has slowed but her smile is bigger than ever. Glancing down at her purple shoes, I remember the day she bought them at Ready to Run in Austin. Modeling them for me in our living room, the smile on her face and the care she took tying them reminded me of a kid who had just gotten her first bike. *These* were her shoes for *New York*!

She has worn them faithfully and they have served her well for countless miles.

I think of the miles ahead.

3

SPIRITUALLY MUDDLED

HIDING

With a petite frame and straight dark brown hair that reaches past her shoulders, she appears to be in her early thirties. Wearing jeans, a lightweight gray cardigan sweater, and blue Adidas running shoes, an inviting smile shapes her face and pushes against her natural shyness. Not long after she takes her seat next to my daughter, Holly, I learn that her name is Deena.

She, her husband, and their two young children sit across the jumbo jet's aisle from my family: Tracey, my wife; our daughters, Meredith and Holly, ages eleven and nine; and me. All of us are heading to Italy.

On the long, overnight flight to Rome, Deena and I have several brief interactions between our attempts at getting some sleep. Holly finally nods off with her head in my lap and her gradually unfolding legs encroaching on Deena, who gives a maternal "it's OK" wave as she slowly closes her own eyes.

At one point in the flight, I notice that her hands shake rather vigorously. They don't shake when at rest in her lap or on her seatback tray, which would be typical for Parkinson's disease, but rather when she tries to use them, such as when opening a packet of peanuts or holding her fork; or when she changes TV channels on the touchscreen monitor built into the seatback in front of her. I see Holly glancing at her hands several times and then quickly looking away. With my peripheral vision, I can see her struggling to steady her reach and I watch her almost constantly for several hours. As sleepy as I am, I cannot close my eyes.

At several junctures, she sighs, and at one point, she slams a pack of crackers down after several attempts to open them. I want to offer to help, and even more to ask about her condition.

I noticed your hand tremors . . .

This is awkward, but do you have essential tremor? Or is it Parkinson's disease?

. . . Because, well, I have it.

But I never say a word.

SEARCHING

It's the summer of 2017, about eight months after my Parkinson's diagnosis. Only Tracey, my doctors, and three or four close friends know I have this disease. Otherwise, I'm carrying the burden of secrecy.

For several years, Tracey and I had planned to take the girls to Europe. But it was one of the things we'd put off. We told ourselves it would be expensive, and the girls would get more out of the trip and remember it more vividly when they were older. We assumed we had unlimited time.

We land in Rome at around 10 AM on a Sunday morning and go directly to the apartment we rented in Trastevere, a vibrant and eclectic neighborhood located on the Tiber River, west of Rome's center and just south of Vatican City.

I take off my shoes in the apartment's front portico, and the cool ceramic tile floor soothes my warm feet. As I pull two of our four carry-on roller suitcases through the minimalist living area, my eyes lock on the stainless steel moka pot—a stovetop espresso maker—prominently displayed on the kitchen counter. Tracey's Italian grandparents always had one, which they often used for making "the black coffee" after dinner.

Immaculate and quiet, the apartment opens up beyond the kitchen to a courtyard with dozens of flowers in bloom. Pinks and yellows, purples and oranges invite unanticipated joy and calm. A fresh mixed-flower bouquet sits on a small black wrought iron table that looks newly painted with two matching chairs. The bouquet blows in the gentle wind, keeping pace with the matching contents of small rectangular terra-cotta flower boxes placed in each of four windowsills.

Exhausted after the long flight, we prepare to settle in and take a brief nap.

"I think it's time to spray the bidet and hit the hay!" Meredith says.

Later that afternoon, we head to Vatican City.

SEEKING

For several miles, he's engaged us in rapid conversation about various things Roman—places to see, museums to visit, food to eat. The small-framed, middle-aged taxi driver has big white teeth and jet-black hair. He offers a pleasant "arrivederci" before stopping the car and letting the four of us out a few blocks from Vatican City's outer wall. As the warm sun shines brightly, we walk toward St. Peter's Square on narrow gray brick roads called sampietrini. Tracey gasps over the architectural beauty while Meredith, Holly, and I breathe in the smells of garlic and al fresco dining that waft in the air. All of us are hungry, so we stop to have dinner at La Vittoria, which a family friend had recommended.

Seated on the front patio, we eat pasta and pizza and sip wine as the ends of red gingham tablecloths move with the gentle breeze. The red matches my bloodshot eyes, as I did not sleep on the flight from the states the night before. I watch scores of people—locals, tourists, and religious pilgrims—scurrying over sidewalks and crosswalks as they go about their business. Motorized scooters that outnumber cars weave through the thickening traffic in seemingly choreographed ways. An occasional horn interrupts the otherwise low, steady hum of city life.

After dinner and a stop at the impressive gelato counter a few doors away, we continue the walk to St. Peter's Square. I first glimpse the majestic white stone columns, or colonnades, that wrap around it when walking up a street called Via delle Fornaci, which narrows and becomes Piazza del Sant'uffizio a few hundred feet before you get to the square. Shaped actually more like a circle, the expansive, open space funnels large crowds and one's attention west, toward St. Peter's Basilica, the largest church in the world. Designed in part by Michelangelo, it overlooks the square, where the pope presides periodically at large masses. Some of them draw over 300,000 visitors.

As we cross through the colonnades and walk into the square, the girls take off running across its weathered gray cobblestone pavers. They run first to the Bernini Fountain, the newer of two magnificent fountains in the square, and it is all they can do to refrain from hopping the low steel fencing that encloses it. It's still warm outside and, though a breeze continues to blow, they long to feel the water's coolness.

"Can we get in?" Meredith asks as she flashes a signature mischievous smile. Her olive skin, a gift from Tracey, glows beautifully in the sunlight and fits the Mediterranean surroundings perfectly. "Not unless you want to spend the night in a Vatican jail," I say. Holly lifts her eyebrows, opens her delicious Milk Dud eyes wide, and chuckles.

Not yet twelve, Meredith nevertheless rolls her eyes in that preteen way, and then she and Holly pull away and dart to the tall Obelisk located at the midpoint of the square. Made of granite, and brought to Rome from Egypt by the emperor Caligula in the first century, its four-sided structure rests on four couchant lions and narrows at the top, where it reaches eighty-four feet into the air and is capped by an iron cross that can be seen from a distance. As an ancient pagan monument located in the holiest of Christian settings, it symbolizes humanity reaching out to Christ.[1]

It also functions as a sundial, and as the sun begins to set, it casts growing shadows over the venerable, expansive space.

Tracey continues walking toward the Obelisk, trying to catch up with Meredith and Holly, but I linger behind, drawn in by the fountain's serenity. As Holly turns around to wait for Tracey, the giant dimples in her cheeks, a gift from me, reveal an innocent joy that perhaps only children know. Her flawless skin, protected by a heavy dose of sunblock, still glistens in the evening light.

Turning back toward the fountain, I watch the water spray firmly upward into a sky painted with bold yellow and orange streaks, before reversing course and cascading over two large rounded tiers and back into the ground-level pool. I stand before it for several minutes, soothed by its sounds and occasional wind-blown mist. With its massive and meticulously kept dome, the grand Basilica serves as an inspiring backdrop. The 140 saints, cast in stone and perched atop the wrapping colonnade, add religious heft, while the developmentally delayed young girl in a wheelchair and the middle-aged blind man standing across the pool add humanity.

I stand there thinking about my spiritual path—from attending Duke Divinity School and Princeton Seminary, to spending nearly twenty years as a minister and seminary professor—and I wonder what I really believe.

Why so much suffering and despair in life?

---

1. See http://stpetersbasilica.info/Docs/seminarians.htm#Obelisk.

Why so much injustice and inequity?

Is this all there is?

Jesus said, "Come to me all who labor and who carry heavy burdens, and I will give you rest," and, speaking to his followers for the last time, "Remember, I am with you always, even to the end of the age."

Is this true?

Or did Nietzsche have it right? That, "to live is to suffer and to survive is to find meaning in the suffering"?

Could both be speaking truth?

Will I find something that gives me lasting comfort and hope as the Parkinson's clock ticks?

My eyes flit to the four or five others flanking the fountain, and I wonder if they are exploring similar questions shaped by their own unique circumstances and experiences. Questions having to do with God's existence and power, with God's mercy and concern. Questions I began asking years before and to which I thought I had at least some provisional answers.

With tears falling down my cheeks, I ask God to help me find peace and to preserve my health. Looking beyond the fountain once again, I catch a glimpse of my girls lost in play around the Obelisk, and I ask God to provide for their needs, too, and for Tracey's, and for my parents'. I also ask for the gift of watching Meredith and Holly grow up, and of being active with them; and to be able to write and teach for many years; and to keep making love to my wife; and to still matter, to others and to myself.

. . . And to be an old man when I die.

I want to bathe my face with the cool water.

4

A STRONGER VOICE

VOICE CHANGES

Like many things Parkinsonian, the changes came on slowly and subtly but they did not relent. After a morning of teaching or when speaking a lot at meetings, my throat felt scratchy and sounded tired. Though I had been a public speaker for decades, speaking loudly enough for others to hear me, especially in noisy places, became more challenging and even painful. When I didn't speak from deep in my diaphragm, my conversation partners would say "Huh?" and "What?" more often than ever before, cuing me to repeat more loudly what I had just said.

Many people with Parkinson's experience voice changes. Looking back, my own voice began changing several years before my diagnosis. Since then, I have worked with an exceptional speech therapist named Stephanie Coker, who gives me exercises to help strengthen my voice and coaches me on how I may use it differently.

VOICE CHALLENGES

Late one Wednesday morning, in the spring of 2017, I still have not shared my diagnosis beyond three or four close friends. I stand in front of a group of first-year University of Texas students in a course I teach in the Steve Hicks School of Social Work. Titled *Mentoring Boys into Men*, the course focuses on male psychological and social development, or psychosocial development in social work speak.

As we cover the day's topic, I speak about the pressures that boys and men face, beginning at very young ages, to conform to norms of masculinity, norms that discourage emotional vulnerability, intimacy, and connection.

"These pressures and norms are not only unhelpful but, in most cases, they're unnatural and unattainable," I say. "From the time they're born, we teach boys to push against what's natural. We discourage them from showing any vulnerability, much less weakness, which, of course, we often equate. The same goes for intimacy and authentic human connections; we do not encourage this either. Instead, we teach and reward boys and men for independence, stoicism, and endurance. We teach them to lead isolated lives, emotionally cut off from themselves and others, especially when they are in pain. For boys and men, anger is often the only emotion that we allow and validate."

After pausing for a moment, I ask, "So, how do you see this changing?"

One of the students, a young Middle Eastern woman, Aisha, raises her hand.

I nod for her to speak.

"We need to call on adults, and especially men, to help break the cycle," she says, "and that can happen only when more men risk speaking up about their true feelings and also display different behaviors tied to different norms of masculinity."

I smile as she continues, a lump forming in my throat.

"We need men to be more vulnerable, to show strength by taking risks that may make them seem weak, at least to themselves, but actually make them strong—strong because it makes them human. As a society, we should applaud when men admit their fears, when they face them, head on, and ask others to support them. This is how deeper and more authentic connections form, and it's the only way things will change."

She speaks all of this from the front row, with an adolescent's conviction and middle-aged wisdom.

"Thank you. I couldn't agree with you more," I say.

As the words leave my mouth, I clasp my hands firmly in front of me, to camouflage the back-and-forth shudder of my tremoring index finger. Then, walking across the wide and shallow classroom and listening to other students' responses, I place my hand in my pocket to hide my stiff, bent Parkinson's elbow.

"HEY YOU"

A few days later, at a bus stop on campus, I meet James.

He has short hair, a full beard, and wears faded baggy jeans, black high-top sneakers, and a red hoodie. I assume he is in his early twenties. With a single earbud, he listens to something on his phone, and with his right index and middle fingers, he taps on a tattered blue notebook opened in his lap. Walking closer, I can hear the rhythms of a hip-hop beat. It sounds familiar, but I cannot quite make it out. Playing with words, James sounds out different lyrics before vigorously writing them down. None of the dozens of people walking by seem to notice, much less to care.

I interrupt.

"May I ask what you're working on?" I say.

He looks up from his notebook and squints, his head cocked slightly to the side.

After a brief hesitation, he says, "I'm sounding out raps to a beat. Here . . . have a listen."

Unplugging the earbud from his phone, he turns up the volume. Now, I recognize the song—"Hey You," by Pink Floyd.

"That's a great song . . . it's been around a long time . . . and I like what you're doing with it," I say. "I've been listening to you and your words are powerful."

He looks at me with slightly more squinted eyes, as if to further hone his bullshit detector. I worry that I have said the wrong thing.

He continues to stare before offering a slight nod and a half smile.

"My raps aren't about getting more things, or being violent, or objectifying people, man. I'm bipolar, and I rap about that," he says.

I nod and wait for him to continue.

"I try to be a voice for voiceless people, man. You know, people who live with depression, schizophrenia, and other kinds of mental illness. We are usually ignored, or misunderstood. You feel me?"

"I do . . . and . . . and I'm sorry," I say. "It shouldn't be this way."

He does not say anything but purses his lips and offers another half nod, his eyes now scanning me.

"I'm Allan," I say.

"James, bro," he says.

We shake hands.

"Can I ask you something else, James?"

"Shoot," he says.

"What can someone like me do to help change that?"

"Just don't be silent, man. Speak up! 'Cause people will listen to you," he says.

Swallowing hard, I clear my scratchy throat.

"Thank you. That's good advice," I say.

He keeps looking at me. I try not to avert my eyes.

"Don't be silent, man," he says again.

My bus pulls up; its squeaking brakes intrude.

"I hear you, James, and I'm glad we met."

He gives me a fist bump, reinserts the earbud, and looks back at his blue notebook.

***

I am still learning from Stephanie. I am also learning how to take the kinds of risks that Aisha called for, and, like James, how to speak with a stronger voice.

5

CRAFTING A PARKINSON'S STORY

A NEUROLOGIST

"I want you to remember something. It's really important. People experience this disease differently. It's not the same for everyone." Dr. T, my diagnosing neurologist, then pauses, looks me in the eye, and with a Texan's directness and authenticity says, "Don't let someone else's story become your story."

A CRAFTSMAN

The summer after that fateful fall meeting with Dr. T, my wife, Tracey, our daughters, Meredith and Holly, and I make a trip to Rome. On the sidewalk in the Trastevere neighborhood, just outside our rented apartment's front door, I watch a small, older Italian man working methodically to install something in an adjacent apartment. Made of ornamental iron, it looks like a portion of a decorative handrail for a staircase, or perhaps a piece of a light fixture.

I can't tell for sure.

Barely five feet tall and stocky, he works from a tiny car, using the small hatchback area and the sidewalk as his workstation. Many Romans drive small cars, especially when compared to what typical Americans drive. In fact, other than government vehicles, I don't recall seeing an SUV anywhere in Italy. This man works from a dark gray Fiat with black interior, which he's squeezed into a parking space that's only a fraction larger than the car.

His Fiat holds various tools and supplies, including a small saw that he uses to cut several pieces of iron, and a stationary file, which he uses to shape it. The file sits in a vice atop a pop-up workbench he's placed on the sidewalk, just above a small gas generator that powers his saw. A stainless steel utility bucket also rests on the ground, next to the workbench, and holds additional tools. The large pocket attached to his leather tool belt has still more tools in it, and from its side hangs a cloth rag, a tape measure, and a small flashlight.

A minimalist by nature, I admire his efficiency and economy of space; how he gets so much work done with so few tools. Trying to remain unnoticed, I watch him work for at least ten minutes.

He takes several pieces of iron from his car, judges whether or not they fit together correctly, and on more than one occasion he measures them. He then cuts some of the pieces and begins a shaping and fitting process. He cuts the iron, bends it into form, files its edges, and rubs it smooth with the rag on his tool belt. Wiping his sweaty hands across the bottom of a worn and stained apron, he walks with a significant limp and labors when bending the down to retrieve a tool from his bucket.

As his design takes shape, he blows residual metal shards off it with quick bursts of air from his mouth. It sounds like he has an air compressor in his chest. The smells of hot metal waft by, colliding with hints of garlic and smoked meat. My eyes stay locked on this metallurgic maestro, who never glances away from his creation.

A DESIGNER

After a few days in Rome, we take the train to Florence, where we have rented an apartment that overlooks the Arno River. Across the street from our apartment, there is a public access beach and outdoor bar, which I take note of and plan to visit one evening.

The next day, after hours of visiting museums, churches, and gelato bars, we walk along the south bank of the river toward our apartment. Meredith spots a lot of commotion on the beach and up and down the long inclined driveway providing access to it. As we approach, we see a growing group of people lining the rock wall that overlooks the beach and driveway, and when we stop to ask what's going on, we learn that a well-known Italian children's clothing brand, Il Gufo, is about to have a fashion show.

Now, I don't know Il Gufo from Gap Kids, but it quickly becomes clear that we will be staying to watch this fashion show, from start to finish, and that the cold beer I have my heart set on will have to wait.

The sun begins to set, and dozens of people begin making their way from a parking lot located on the street level, to the security checkpoint adjacent to the outdoor bar. Then, they walk down the long descending driveway and into the area of the beach where the fashion show will take place. Each person who passes below us could have leapt off a magazine page—with beautiful clothes, coiffed hair, straight teeth, unblemished skin, no gray hair, presumably big bank accounts, and otherwise seemingly perfect lives.

But, of course, there are no perfect lives. As Anne Lamott says, all of us have to learn to dance with a limp.

Those in the growing crowd walk leisurely toward portable grandstands that back up to the wall over which we are looking, and that have turned the beach area into an amphitheater. Many of them stop several times to chat along the way.

At one point, I notice a parting of the crowd gathered at the top of the driveway, just before the security checkpoint. A dark blue Mercedes sedan makes its way slowly toward the beach, and a few people wave as it passes them. It has tinted windows, so I cannot see who is inside. I assume it's a designer, or maybe a celebrity spokesperson for the brand, or perhaps an executive with Il Gufo. Whatever, it is someone with stature and influence in that industry.

The car stops in a staging area just beyond where the props for the fashion show end—it's a Polynesian-themed set—and a cargo van, which had been parked close by, pulls up beside it. Four men exit quickly and walk with purpose to the van's back doors, which open to its cargo area. They begin taking out flat and rectangle-shaped folding stainless steel squares and place them in the sand beside the driver's door. They work quickly but calmly. As these squares begin to take the form of a longer line, I can see that they are assembling a sidewalk. By now, portable lights that reach high in the air on both sides of the grandstands are on, casting an almost fluorescent glow over the entire scene.

The driver's door is now open, and I see a handsome man, who appears to be in his late fifties, waiting patiently in his seat. Every few seconds he turns his head to the right, speaking to someone who has come with him to the show. I cannot see the person clearly, but it appears to be a woman with long dark hair. Occasionally, the man glances in his side mirror to observe the sidewalk team at work before turning again to his companion. His tan body and dark, slicked-back hair makes his white linen shirt pop under the lights.

Then, one of the workers opens the trunk of the Mercedes, reaches inside, and removes an all-black wheelchair. He places it on the metal sidewalk and opens it up so that the seat flattens out. He then pushes it to the driver's side door.

By now, the driver's companion has made her way around the car, and, with the wind blowing her hair, she assists him with getting out of the car and into the wheelchair. She is as beautiful and dignified as he is, wearing a floral-patterned sundress and sporting a luxurious brown leather handbag slung across her body. As she pulls her silky hair out of her eyes, I notice several gold bangles on her wrist, and then, a large ring on her left hand, which makes me look at his hands, too. I see him wearing a white gold wedding band, similar to my own.

I wonder how long it has been this way. For him. For her.

She bends down as he says something to her, and then nods her head and smiles. A line of people has formed along the metal sidewalk, almost like a tunnel of friends you see at a wedding, or a group of comrades assembling to touch swords at military parades. She begins to push her husband toward the appreciative crowd as the four men pull away in the cargo van.

I look at Tracey. She smiles at me with a kind of tenderness that's typical for her, but which I've often struggled to receive. I put my arm around her and squeeze her lower back. She puts her arm around me and does the same. A lump sits firmly in my throat.

"Daddy, I think it's about to start," Holly says.

"Finally!" says Meredith.

Music begins playing over a loud speaker.

The four of us take a half step forward and peer over the wall.

HARDSHIPS AND HOPES

Don't let someone else's story become your story.

I appreciate Dr. T's advice, and I recall it often. Though it is difficult for all of us who live with it, the Parkinson's beast affects people differently, and, over time, it can prompt a variety of challenges. Some of them can lead to walking with a limp, others can require the use of a wheelchair, and others might be hidden, such as depression, anxiety, or insomnia. As my friend Michael Westphal put it, "Parkinson's makes you uncomfortable in your own body." Consequently, while no Parkinson's story lacks hardships, these will differ among people.

But I also think a lot about the craftsman and the designer, and about their stories.

With physical challenges and restricted resources, they create beautiful things.

6

TELLING MY PARENTS

How do you tell the people you love most that you have a progressive neurologic disease? Many people with Parkinson's, as well as those with other serious illnesses, struggle with this question. I certainly did. In fact, the two conversations that I most anticipated and dreaded were telling my parents I have Parkinson's and then telling my children.

Here is how it went with my parents.

THE PLAN

It's a Wednesday morning, and I'm with Tracey and our children, in Surfside Beach, South Carolina. As we have done for many years, we met my parents there for a weeklong stay. I spent my high school years just a few miles north, in Myrtle Beach, and although I moved away over thirty years ago, a portion of my soul still lives in that part of the world. Being by the ocean and smelling salty, humid air, if only for one week each year, resets me. It also takes me back to a fondly remembered childhood in coastal South Carolina. If you have ever visited this region or read a Pat Conroy novel, you probably have a sense of its charm.

Tracey has taken the girls to the beach. I hang back to wait for my parents to return from the grocery store. I think back to a day earlier, when speaking by phone with my longtime friend, Elizabeth, with whom I went to college and who lives with her own chronic illness, multiple sclerosis

(MS). Along with neurologic challenges, she and I share a love of writing and we speak often about our respective projects and our journeys with illness. She is a fount of wisdom, not to mention possessing a wicked smart sense of humor, and I had shared news of my diagnosis with her several months earlier.

"It's time," I said. "I have to tell them."

The early morning coastal sun beats down and the air is thick. I smell pine and Coppertone sunscreen as I wipe my sweaty face with a blue bandana.

Hiding my condition from my parents, whom I love so much, weighs on me. It's been nine months, and I feel as though, over time, my secrecy will take more away from me than Parkinson's ever could.

"I get it," Elizabeth told me. "It's tough to carry this . . . and mostly by yourself."

With equal measures of generosity and patience, she listened.

"If it were my child, I would want to know," I confessed.

"Of course. You would want to offer your support."

She echoed what Tracey has said from the beginning.

"It's not fair to them for me to hold this. It's time to have The Talk."

Elizabeth continues to listen and offers more encouragement as I keep trying to psych myself up for one of the two most difficult conversations I have ever had. The other would come a few weeks later, when I tell my children I have Parkinson's.

"I bet it'll help you feel better, too," Elizabeth said. "You've given this a lot of thought."

"You'd make a great social worker," I said.

We both laugh.

She thanks me and says, "Let me know how it goes."

THE TALK

For more than thirty minutes, I pace from one side of our rented beach house to the other. When my parents arrive, I put away groceries, organize things on the countertops, and continue to move around. I walk outside and grab beach towels that we have hung on the balcony to dry. I fold and then refold them, make multiple trips upstairs trying to calm myself, and pee three times.

As I return to the first floor and meander by once again, my father looks at me.

"Are you OK?" he asks.

My mother, who is preparing lunch, looks up and sights me, too.

I pause.

"I want to talk with you about something," I say.

My mother stops what she is doing and moves toward the dining area table, where she and I each take a seat. My father comes closer but remains standing behind her, his hands resting on the back of her chair.

Taking a deep breath, I say, "I need to tell you something, but before I do I want you to know that it's going to be OK."

"Are you sick?" my mother immediately asks, with a tearful expression that captures what I knew was an already breaking heart. Somehow, she knows.

"I have Parkinson's disease," I say.

For a few moments, time and speech slow, like when a boxer takes a blow to the head in the movies. The late morning bright light pushes through the large plate glass window's salty film to illuminate the agony on my mother's face.

"My God," she whispers, covering her mouth with her hand. My father grimaces, and with closed eyes silently shakes his head. I see his grip tighten on the back of the chair, as if he has taken a boxer's blow himself.

"I knew something wasn't right," my mother says. "That's why I asked you if you were OK after that doctor's office called."

She is referring to the time when someone from a medical practice in Houston called my parents looking for one "Allan Cole."

"I'm sorry I didn't tell you the truth," I say.

My dad puts his arm around her and she reaches out to hug me. He puts his other arm around my neck to complete our three-way hug. We hold that comforting position, arm in arm, for a while before we let go and my father sits down.

Then, I slowly take them through the previous months in my Parkinson's story.

I describe my symptoms, multiple doctor's visits, the misdiagnosis, the diagnosis, and the prognosis. They ask a few questions, some of them a couple of times. One of them is if I have any pain, and I assure them I do not. Another question relates to my prognosis. I understand. It takes some time for it all to settle in. Reassuring them reassures me.

I tell them I want to use Parkinson's to do some good, for me, my family, the Parkinson's community, and others. I muse about what forms this good might take, telling them I hope to get involved in education, advocacy, and raising money for Parkinson's research.

As much as anything, I want to be honest with them, to be authentic about my struggles and concerns, to speak realistically about the future. I also want to set a tone of hopefulness and determination. I aim to display a positive attitude about both the present and the future, which I genuinely have and want them to embrace, not just on this day but also in the years to come.

"I'm sorry you have this. I will be strong for you. This will be OK," my mother says.

"We'll take this on as a family," says my father.

We talk for a few more minutes before Tracey and the girls return to the beach house.

A part of me wants my mom and dad to make it all just go away, as they did so many times when I hurt as a child.

THE PATH AHEAD

They cannot make it go away, of course. No one can, as of yet. This may change in my lifetime, and I never discount that possibility, that hope. There are many reasons for hope, including significant scientific progress and new treatments discovered each year. "We know how to treat this disease, and we are on the verge of real breakthroughs," Dr. T, my diagnosing neurologist, told me.

As I wait for that day, along with 10 million others who have Parkinson's and the many millions more who offer them love, support, and encouragement, this is what I know. Removing the freight of going it alone—pallets of secrecy, silence, fear, and shame—is itself life-giving and peace-filled, more than you might ever imagine possible.

Not only this, but daring to lean on those who love you most, and who pledge their abiding presence, will help you, and them, weather many storms, including Parkinson's disease, and in doing so will help you discover new strength.

This strength can prompt a new kind of resolve. The resolve to live each day with more immediacy and gratitude, with a keener awareness of life's fragility and unpredictability, but also its beauty; with an eye newly honed for seeing human suffering and need, and with an unwavering commitment to being present for others while expecting they will be present for you.

I am speaking of the resolve to take on what lies ahead.

Together. Arm in arm. Come what may.

7

TELLING MY CHILDREN

How do you tell the people you love most that you have a progressive neurologic disease? Many people with Parkinson's, and those with other serious illnesses, struggle with this question. I certainly did. In fact, the two conversations that I most anticipated and dreaded were telling my parents I have Parkinson's and then telling my children.

Here is how it went with my kids.

RINGING THE BELL

It's a Saturday morning, ten months after my diagnosis. My wife, Tracey, has just returned from an early run and our daughters are still fast asleep. Holly, who is nine, will likely be up soon. Meredith, our eleven-year-old, will sleep until we force her to get out of bed. The bedroom window is open and an unseasonably cool breeze blows in the sounds of chirping birds. A neighbor's dog yaps in the distance.

I stare at myself in the bathroom mirror. The Texas Longhorns cotton T-shirt that I have slept in, a gift from Tracey and the girls a couple of years earlier, reminds me of less complicated days. Its gray color matches the morning stubble on my face, and its wrinkles correspond with the corners of my eyes that hint at a new kind of sadness carried deep within.

I grab a towel and make the one block walk to my gym. After stretching and doing exercises to improve my balance, I walk toward four rows of treadmills and elliptical machines faced by nearly a dozen television screens. A faint smell of sweat mixed with ammonia hangs in the air. Given my loss of smell, an early Parkinson's symptom, I wonder if it stinks worse than I know.

Before stepping on a treadmill, I speak briefly to a couple of friends I have known for many years. Our kids have grown up together, and they are part of my community. If they knew I have Parkinson's they would be supportive and encouraging, but I have not shared my news.

I slide my ear buds into my ears, take a drink from my water bottle, and pull up a music playlist on my phone.

After a few minutes on the treadmill, I break a sweat and my lungs have expanded. When I find my running cadence, the song "Box of Rain" by the Grateful Dead begins to play. It has been a favorite of mine since I first heard it at Davidson College in the late eighties. When I hear it now, it takes me back to when it played over and over again on my roommate's Pioneer turntable in Belk Hall. The hallway outside our room often smelled like sweat, too, absent ammonia but with an old beer and cold pizza overlay.

As I run, my body glossy with sweat and my breathing getting quicker, I hear the band's bassist, Phil Lesh, sing about the power of love to get you through life's difficulties—to "see you through."

Tears begin to fall over my cheekbones as my thoughts flash back to the last year of my life, and I linger there for a moment. Bone-chilling sadness, fear, so many questions, and an enormous sense of loss have swallowed me. These feelings have ebbed and flowed since those early weeks and months after the diagnosis, but they still visit occasionally. I imagine they always will.

I reach for my towel and wipe the sweaty tears from my face, and then take another drink from my water bottle, which my girls typically use for school and which has red, pink, and purple hearts all around it.

My thoughts jump to what going public with my Parkinson's will be like, and how life will be different once people know. "You can't un-ring that bell," I frequently say to Tracey.

Who will pity or dismiss me? Who will treat me differently or think I have lost too much to matter any longer? Who will never acknowledge that I have Parkinson's, whether because they're uncomfortable or because they don't care? For the better part of a year, these fears have nearly paralyzed me. I have spent so much energy speculating and worrying.

You are still the same Allan, Tracey keeps saying, *our friends will be sources of support.*

I also know that my secret has become too much to bear.

My mind fixes on Meredith and Holly, and on how I want them to see me, their father, live authentically, face adversity, and try to make something good spring from it.

I want them to know the truth.

DOPA WHAT?

I finish my workout and walk home from the gym. After taking a quick shower, I join Tracey, Holly, and Meredith in our living room. The girls sit on the floor drawing in their sketchbooks. Tracey sits on the sofa, bookended by our two sleeping dogs, Sunny and Fiona. I take a seat across from Tracey, in the recliner. Soft music plays in the background. It's an uncharacteristically mellow moment in our home.

Holly crawls up into my lap, bringing her sketchbook with her. Her hair smells like cookies and shampoo. Meredith remains on the floor hard at work. The tip of her tongue sticks out from her mouth.

Not knowing how to begin, I mention a close friend who lives with a chronic disease, noting her recent struggles.

"It must be really hard for her," Meredith says.

I try to calm my quivering voice.

"I think you're right, Mer. But having the love of her family and friends probably helps a lot," I say.

After a brief silence, I get up my nerve.

"I wanted you girls know that I'm living with a disease," I say.

"What?" Meredith says, with her big brown Milk Dud eyes opened wide. "What do you mean?"

Holly looks up at me, too, with puffy, poked-out lips.

"Daddy! What disease?" she asks.

Taking a deep breath, I say, "I have something called Parkinson's disease."

My bottom lip begins to quiver.

Don't you cry, I say to myself.

"Are you going to die, Daddy?" Holly asks, her eyes now growing moist.

"No, honey, you don't die from Parkinson's. It's something I can live with for a long time."

"But that's an old person's disease, Daddy, and you're not old," Meredith says. ". . . *Oh my God*, I don't want you walking with a cane."

"Not everyone with Parkinson's needs a cane, Mer . . . and you're right, most people who get Parkinson's are older; but not *everyone* is older when they get it. Like Michael J. Fox; he got it in his late twenties," I say.

"Who's Michael J. Fox?" Holly asks.

I see Tracey smile.

"He's a famous actor," I say. "He got Parkinson's as a young man; and he's had it a long time; and he's done amazing work raising money to help find better treatments and even a cure; and he's taught us a lot about how to live a good life with this disease."

Tracey's kind eyes urge me on.

"I'm not going to die from Parkinson's, but over time, probably after many years, it's going to get harder for me to move. I will probably get slower and stiffer, and my hands might begin to shake a little. Most people with Parkinson's have these kinds of symptoms at some point," I say.

"What causes it, Daddy?" Holly asks, pulling her lips into her mouth and biting down, her eyes shining from moisture.

"There's a chemical in your brain called dopamine, which helps send signals to your body so that it can move the right way. When you have Parkinson's, you are losing dopamine, and, over time, it gets harder for your body to do what your brain wants it to do. It gets harder to move," I say.

"Dopa what?" Holly asks.

"I've heard of dopamine," Meredith says. "But how long have you known this?"

She's now glaring at me, her eyes looking more like brown darts.

"I've known since last fall," I say.

"*What?* You've known *that* long? Why did you wait to tell us?" Meredith says. "I'm mad about that. We are old enough for you to tell us these things. Daddy, I wish you'd told me."

Her voice cracks.

Holly looks back at me. She still has tears in her eyes.

"It's going to be OK, honey. My doctors tell me I'm going to be OK for a long time; and there are good medicines available now, and others will be coming out in the next few years. It's going to be OK."

Trying her best not to cry, Holly asks, "Can we still go to Disney?"

She is referring to plans we made to go with my mom and dad to Disney World in the spring.

"Of course, my love. We are going to have a great trip. And we are going to have a great life, with many more fun trips ahead," I say.

She gives me a hug and then gets back on the floor to resume drawing.

"I'm mad, Daddy. You should have told us," Meredith says.

"I'm sorry you're angry, Mer. I needed some time to learn more about Parkinson's and to get more comfortable with having it. I didn't want you and Holly to worry."

"But you should have told us. Or, at least you should have told *me*; I'm old enough," she says.

"I'm sorry. I told you when I was ready. I hope you'll forgive me and understand," I say, as I get on the floor and kiss her on the head.

"I forgive you, Daddy, but you still should have told us," she says with a mischievous smirk.

I get up from the floor and walk to the back of the house and into the bathroom. Looking into the mirror, my eyes well up yet again. I exhale and wash my face. A few minutes later, I go back into the living room, where my three loves still sit.

"Who wants breakfast tacos?" I ask.

"Duh," Meredith says. "When do I *not* want breakfast tacos?"

"I want some, too, Daddy," Holly says.

"I'll have one," says Tracey.

We often have breakfast tacos on the weekends. Basically, this is a family ritual that most Texans will understand. Much of the time, the girls posture for their preferred source. Holly likes Taco Shack, while Meredith always lobbies for Torchy's. There is none of their arguing this morning. They each put in their orders, their usual requests. Meredith wants sausage and egg; Holly, potato and cheese; and Tracey, egg and cheese.

As I get to the front door, Meredith says, "One more thing Daddy, you should order the dopamine taco special."

8

TELLING MY BOSS

NAMING MY FEARS

It's Tuesday morning, a few minutes before a standing 10 o'clock meeting with my boss, and my heart beats quickly as I walk back to my office after a third trip to the bathroom. I have rehearsed the conversation I am about to have with him dozens of times. How I'd let him know about my having Parkinson's disease. It has been nearly a year since I found out.

Wanting to understand my rights and the university's obligations, I consulted with an employment attorney who told me the law was on my side. I had no rational reason for thinking otherwise, for feeling so vulnerable. I was treated fairly and was confident that would continue. Still, I was afraid.

I did not fear losing my job. My fear rested with the possibility of losing a reputation twenty years in the making, as a scholar, teacher, and administrator, and in a university that I have loved since my childhood in Plano, Texas. Rather, I feared losing the confidence of my boss, colleagues, and students; losing opportunities to grow and advance; and losing my standing in what I have long understood to be my calling in life.

Many people are naïve about Parkinson's, including highly educated people; they make misassumptions about what those who have it can and cannot do. This is why many of us, at least for a while, choose to stay silent.

LOOKING FOR GUIDANCE

I took some cues from my friend Bret Parker, who learned he has Parkinson's in 2007, at the age of thirty-eight. An accomplished attorney, he heads the New York City Bar Association as its Executive Director. To disclose his illness he wrote a piece for *Forbes* titled "The Last Workplace Secret."[1]

Bret understood both the professional and social risks that come when one lives publicly with a disease like Parkinson's, and he labored for five years before telling people he had it. I could understand his waiting.

I read Bret's piece not long after my diagnosis, when I combed the Internet day and night for information about Parkinson's and for personal accounts of those living with it. Wanting desperately to find people living a good life, an active and meaningful life with Parkinson's, I found hope in Bret's story.

It would be several more months until we met and before I was ready to follow his lead, but Bret's honesty and courage inspired and equipped me for revealing my own secret. Through his efforts to raise awareness and money for Parkinson's research, he inspires me still.

REFINING MY PURPOSE

I wanted to use my condition to make a difference, and to connect with others living with Parkinson's, and to build relationships through our shared challenges. I wanted to get going on all of this, and soon. But before I could do this I had some serious internal work to do on myself. It was ironic, really. Before Parkinson's, I thought I had my life's biggest questions figured out. Maybe I had for a time, but this was a new life with a wrinkle, a twist, a curve ball. This new life required a close, second look.

David Brooks has said, "We are all fragile when we don't know what our purpose is, when we haven't thrown ourselves with abandon into a social role, when we haven't committed ourselves to certain people, when we feel like a swimmer in an ocean with no edge. . . . People are really tough only after they have taken a leap of faith for some truth or mission or love. Once they've done that they can withstand a lot."[2]

I had lived contently for many years with satisfactory answers to questions about resilience (what Brooks calls "toughness"), my life's purpose,

1. Parker, "Parkinson's Disease."
2. Brooks, "Making Modern Toughness."

and my personal commitments; but my diagnosis brought many seemingly settled questions to the forefront of my consciousness. I liken the reemergence of these big questions after Parkinson's—deep, existential, and pressing—to what you hear people say about a midlife crisis. In both cases, you consider whom you have been and whom you want to be.

Before getting Parkinson's, I had spent much of my professional life thinking, teaching, and writing about resilience and purpose. I urged my students to explore the big questions for themselves, those having to do with who they are, what they believe, and what they are called to do. Seeking my own answers and helping others find theirs has shaped my self-understanding and sense of purpose for as long as I can remember. Still, despite this personal history, when I found out I have Parkinson's I felt like that swimmer in "an ocean with no edge." More accurately, I felt as if I was not swimming so much as trying to tread water. To locate that edge, that guiding boundary, I needed to reexamine things like my ideas about right and wrong, as well as things such as how I spend my time to maximize fulfillment and joy. I had to reevaluate almost everything, even as I sought to rely on my "toughness" and renewed commitments to living out higher yearnings.

Eventually, I began to feel like I had new perspectives to draw on, those tied to living with a progressive and incurable disease. I had new insights about hope, will, purpose, competence, fidelity, love, care, and wisdom. Sharing these insights and helping others explore and answer their own questions, to find their own guiding boundary in an ocean that threatens to swallow them, became my goal. Parkinson's had become my teacher, and I wanted to share what I was learning with others. That desire gave rise to my creating a blog, PD Wise (PDWise.com), among other efforts to use the Parkinson's beast for something good.

YOU DO YOU

Few decisions are more personal than disclosing a medical diagnosis, particularly at work, and especially one that drastically changes your life and risks altering the way others look at you and your future. *I would never suggest that anyone should disclose on any timeline other than a personal one.* Some people need to speak publicly about their Parkinson's immediately. Others wait a decade or longer. Some never disclose. Just as the disease presents differently in people, with varying symptoms and degrees of difficulty, and just as it progresses in different ways and at differing rates, so does readiness to speak about it with others. You will never find a one-size-fits-all approach.

I waited nearly eleven months before I went public. While I would describe myself as a private person, keeping the secret eventually became too painful. The agony of its ache far exceeded the effects of the disease itself. Keeping the secret also prevented me from doing things I wanted to do, for myself, my children, and on behalf of those living with Parkinson's and other chronic illnesses. More important, keeping the secret meant lying to people I love, and who love me. Secrets maintain enormous power over those who hold them. Over time, their power can prove destructive.

WORK TO BE DONE

Getting back to the meeting with my boss . . .

We have exhausted the agenda when I say, "Luis, I need to share something with you. It's personal . . . and I am going to try not to cry."

His look of curiosity quickly elides into concern as I take a deep breath.

"Last October, I found out I have Parkinson's disease . . ."

My voice cracks.

"Take your time," he says.

After another deep breath, I walk him through the first symptoms, the weeks of waiting after a misdiagnosis, the DaTscan, the whole story up to this point. He listens patiently, nods, and urges me along with kindness and grace. He asks a few questions, which I answer, and offers words of support that will remain between the two of us.

Looking around his office, and seeing his shelves full of books, a framed *New York Times* op-ed he had written several years earlier, and a Texas Longhorns football helmet signed by players and coaches, I felt more grateful than ever to do this work . . . in this place . . . with these people.

When the conversation ends, we stand up from the table, and shake hands as we slap each other on the back with a half hug. As I turn toward the door he says, "One more thing, Allan. You might have to remind me about your having Parkinson's. We'll both be busy; we've got a lot of work to do." It is exactly what I need to hear.

9

FROM SILENCE TO FREEDOM

SILENCE

One evening, I walk quietly into our dining room where my backpack rests in a chair. I keep a bottle of Azilect in it, a first-line Parkinson's medication that I started when my doctor diagnosed me. Unzipping the lower front pocket, I grab the small white plastic bottle with a bright blue label, shake out a single pill, and put it in my mouth.

"Daddy, are you OK?" my nine-year-old daughter Holly asks.

A sensitive and perceptive child, I wonder if she knows something is amiss.

My wife Tracey and I have discussed when we will tell Holly and her eleven-year-old sister, Meredith, about my Parkinson's; but I am not yet close to being ready. I can hardly tell this new truth to myself.

"I'm fine, Honey. I'm . . . uh . . . I'm just taking something for my allergies," I say.

My heart sinks. The little pill sticks to the lump in my throat.

WORRY

Later that night, after everyone goes to bed, I sit in our living room nursing a beer. After a few minutes of staring at nothing in a dim light, I turn on a lamp and begin looking at books I have on disability, which I have brought home from my campus office. I teach budding social workers, some of whom will work with disabled people of all ages and in many different settings.

Flipping through one of the book's pages, my anxious mind becomes stuck on the prospects of my girls growing up with a declining, and at some point, disabled, dad. I wonder how they will feel about that, and whether I will keep up with their active lives.

As Parkinson's takes a firmer hold on my brain, and my body stiffens and quivers, will I embarrass them?

How will my illness affect them emotionally?

Will I watch them finish college, or get married, or have children from a wheelchair?

Will I be able to provide for their college education, and for other wants and needs?

These questions, and others, haunt me. I still have so much to learn about Parkinson's.

DISGUST

A chapter in one of the books I am looking through speaks of the fear, and even aversion, that some people have toward those with an illness or disability, and of how that may result in their feeling isolated and rejected. Reading to the end of the first page, my blood pressure rising, I take a deep breath and let out a long expletive as I throw the book across the room.

During this same time, I also read Michael Kinsley's book *Old Age: A Beginner's Guide*.[1] He recounts his own experience with Parkinson's disease, which began at age forty-three. I watched him on CNN's *Crossfire* during my college years and appreciated both his keen intellect and his feistiness, which he demonstrated by going toe-to-toe each night with the formidable Pat Buchanan.

Kinsley recalls a dinner party when, seeing his hands shaking, a well-meaning woman offered to cut his steak for him. I cannot bear the thought of someone infantilizing me in such a way, which follows being moved over to the "disabled" column in the social and professional ledgers, and, too often, leads to being written off.

Another's infirmity can make us feel uncomfortable. Discomfort can lead to avoidance.

1. Kinsley, *Old Age*.

SHAME

Those living with illness or disability may practice avoidance, too. Weeks later, I sit in my living room again, this time with a laptop. Tracey is out for an early morning run and the girls have not yet gotten up for school. I pop in my earbuds and hit the play button to watch a video on YouTube. The softness of my recliner folds around me, contrasting with the hard edge against my soul.

As the video begins, a renowned neurologist speaks about his experience with treating Parkinson's disease. "I have many patients who feel ashamed to have the disease," he says. "I tell them, you've done nothing wrong that caused you to have it. It is not something you get because you make poor lifestyle choices or engage in high-risk behaviors. It just happens, and for reasons we still don't know."[2]

Whether due to shame, fear, or other reasons, too many of us live with Parkinson's in secrecy, with anger, and in self-imposed isolation, often until we can no longer hide physical symptoms.

As a result, we suffer in silence.

Alone.

In some cases, for years.

RISK

We need not punish ourselves in this way, and we do not have to carry this extra burden. Telling others what we are facing, including its challenges and our fears, disgust, or shame, even if just a handful of trusted companions or, perhaps, a single one, can prove freeing. Sure, disclosing our condition comes with risks—socially, professionally, and, sometimes, in our most personal relationships. I would never disregard these risks or minimize their potential impact. Telling someone about any hard news, whether Parkinson's-related or otherwise, best happens when it feels right to *oneself*, and never on a one-size-fits-all schedule.

Even so, carrying secrets affects us, too. Silent suffering takes its own destructive toll.

---

2. Many scientists link Parkinson's disease to a genetic predisposition and exposure to certain pesticides. Other risk factors include repeated head trauma, such as occurs in certain sports.

FREEDOM

It took me nearly a year to share my diagnosis publicly, and I wish I had done so sooner. The extraordinary people in my life—some of whom I've met *because* I have Parkinson's, others of whom I've known for years if not forever—were ready to stand and walk with me on this new path; and they haven't missed a single step.

Others who have Parkinson's and who suffered in silence have told me they wish they had risked sharing their diagnosis sooner, too.

After all, there is comfort in not having to hide.

The writer C. S. Lewis put it this way: "I have learned . . . that while those who speak about one's miseries usually hurt, those who keep silence hurt more."[3] There is freedom in living our truth.

3. Lewis, "To Sir Henry Willink," 483.

10

FRIENDSHIP

OLD FRIENDS

"Are you in any pain?" he asks, his eyes opened wide and his body bent slightly forward in the passenger's seat of my car.

Tom and I have known each other for more than thirty years. Having met at Davidson College in 1986, we now live in Austin with our families. We are much closer friends now than we were in college, and I do not recall meeting a kinder or more generous person.

We sit in the Brazos parking garage on the University of Texas campus, having just arrived for the first football game of the 2017 season. It is hot outside, so we welcome the garage's shade and a brisk breeze blowing through it.

My favorite team since childhood and Tom's adopted team, the Texas Longhorns, will play the University of Maryland before a capacity crowd in the iconic Darrell K. Royal Stadium. Each of us sporting customary burnt orange shirts that serve as a Texas fan's uniform, we are prepared.

A POIGNANT CONVERSATION

He asks whether I am in pain because I have just told him about my Parkinson's disease. Other than my wife, Tracey, and my parents, hardly anyone knows what I carry deep within me, namely, the diagnosis that has irreversibly jarred my life. It has been nearly a year, and I still strangle when trying to speak this new truth.

"I don't really have any pain," I say, "mainly discomfort, with stiffness and slowness on my left side; but things will get worse over time . . . it's progressive."

The corners of his mouth now curved downward, Tom listens and nods along as I speak. A part of me wishes we were thirty years younger and talking about Davidson basketball.

"As you might guess, I worry about the future—and especially about parenting Meredith and Holly. They are still so young. I am also anxious about professional implications, even though my doctors tell me I should do well for a long time. And, of course, once people know, you risk them seeing you differently . . . and treating you differently," I say.

I pause. Other than the wind blowing, silence fills the car.

"But I feel so fortunate to have a great wife," I say. "She hasn't wavered in her support and positive outlook; and my parents, they've been amazing. Also, I think the girls will handle it well, once we tell them; and we have a strong community of friends that I can lean on if the need arises," I say.

Speaking these beliefs makes them feel even truer. Calms me, too.

Again, Tom nods. "I'm sorry," he says, "sorry you're facing this."

I then walk him through the last year, from the faint tremor in my left index finger, which sent me to see my doctor, to visits with two neurologists, a DaTscan, and moving conversations with my parents.

He continues to listen, with focused eyes and without interruption.

COMRADES

When I finish, he says, "I'll walk with you on this journey, Allan. Count on me."

I smile and nod.

"But how can I help now?" he says.

I am not sure how to answer him. Still punch drunk from Parkinson's blows, I struggle to find my bearings.

"You're helping already. And I appreciate it," I say. "I'll let you know if there's anything else as I figure more of this thing out. I might need you to talk me off the ledge sometime."

I chuckle. He smiles.

"I'm here for you, brother," he says. "For your family, too . . . and Shelby and our girls will be as well."

"I know. And I'm grateful for that," I say.

We sit there for another moment, and then step out of the car and meet behind it before moving quickly into a handshake that glides into a brief but firm hug and ends with a back slap.

I exhale.

Checking to make sure the tickets are in my shirt pocket, we turn together toward the stadium, where a sea of burnt orange awaits us.

"Hook 'em Horns!" I say.

"Hook 'em!" says Tom.

***

I recall what Ralph Waldo Emerson observed, namely, "It is one of the blessings of old friends that you can afford to be stupid with them."[1]

My friendship with Tom began this way, as being stupid marked too much of my college experience. It's different now. As middle-aged men with wives, daughters, and careers, we navigate the various joys and challenges that inevitably come in this season of life. Too often, we navigate the challenges in silence, and without the help of our friends.

At least I do.

Which is why something else Emerson said rings so true: "A friend is a person with whom I may be sincere. Before [whom] I may think aloud."[2]

---

1. Emerson, *Journals,* 195.
2. Emerson, "Friendship," 119.

11

HUMANIZING WITH HUMOR

DISTRESSING SITUATIONS

With Parkinson's comes emotional distress. It results from biochemical changes in the brain and mainly the loss of dopamine, a neurotransmitter that helps regulate our movement and our mood.

At the same time, certain situations may be particularly distressing.

For instance, those with Parkinson's may have difficulty being with other people who have the disease, at least initially, and especially when others have more advanced Parkinson's and greater impairment. As a friend put it when I encouraged him to attend a local Parkinson's exercise class and support group, "Why would I constantly want to see where I'm headed?"

Another type of stressor comes when seeing people we know for the first time since disclosing our illness publicly, which can make a diagnosis seem more real and lasting, and which may feel awkward to all parties.

I have been in these distressing situations myself.

AHHHHHH!

It's the fall of 2017, nearly a year since my diagnosis but only a few weeks since I revealed it publicly. Peering across the large multipurpose room,

I see people of different ages and at various stages of the disease. I'm the youngest one there by at least ten years. Call me precocious, I guess!

Many in the room shake with hand tremors. A few sit in wheelchairs. Some arrive with the help of a walker. But most seem to function pretty well, or at least well enough to take part in a vigorous workout in hopes of slowing down the Parkinson's beast.

A man named George, whom I had met briefly, catches my eye. In his sixties, noticeably thin, and hunched over in his wheelchair, he appears to have had Parkinson's for many years. He is scrappy, though. I see it in his interactions with those around him, including the instructor. Imagining him as a younger, healthier man, I think about his scrappiness then.

I also wonder if I will share his fate.

It's my first time attending one of the weekly Power for Parkinson's (PFP) exercise classes. Dr. Nina Mosier, PFP's co-founder and president, invited me to try a class after a mutual friend introduced us. Nina and Susan Stahl, her co-founder, became acquainted with Parkinson's disease because their fathers had it, and seeing the benefits of regular exercise and social interaction, as well as the difficulty finding Parkinson's-specific exercise programs, they created Power for Parkinson's, which offers free exercise, dance, and singing classes to people in the Austin area.

Around us, a group of six or eight volunteers, all of them wearing colorful Power for Parkinson's T-shirts, scurry to arrange chairs and to place dumbbells and inflated exercise balls on the floor. Lauren Lewis, a high-energy fitness instructor turned Parkinson's exercise sage, has similarly prepared the area around her, where she will lead the class.

My eyes flit to the far side of the room, where I see our longtime friend and neighbor, Betsy, who, unbeknownst to me, is a PFP volunteer. My quick half-wave meets her surprised look, and as she walks toward me, my heart beats faster and the back of my neck tingles. I also feel hot. It is the first time we have seen each other since I came out of the Parkinson's closet.

We say hello and engage in small talk, and then the awkward silence hits.

"Do you know I have Parkinson's?" I say.

"I just heard that a couple of weeks ago; and I'm sorry . . . but I'm glad you're here."

"Thank you," I say, wondering what else she is thinking.

The class begins, and Lauren leads us through numerous exercises, some while sitting, others while standing, and still others requiring use of the dumbbells or exercise balls. Dance music plays loudly as she counts and directs.

"1–2–3–4, 1–2–3–4. You've got this!" Lauren says.

More than forty of us "Parkies" grind through stiffness, slowness, and tremors to build our core body strength, flexibility, balance, range of motion, and cross-body movements.

"Wooooo!" she yells, the music still blasting.

I see George working hard to keep up.

After nearly an hour, I am sweaty and using muscles I did not know I have.

The music stops, and I hear only the steady hum of the air conditioner. The regulars expect this shift.

"You *all* did great. Now, let's work those voices," Lauren says.

She concludes each class with voice exercises because many people with Parkinson's lose their voice volume and strength.

Following Lauren's commands, we slowly take in a big breath through the nose and then exhale while making the sound "Ahhhhh"—loudly and for as long as we can. It is similar to what you do when visiting the doctor to get your throat looked at.

A symphony of *ahhhhh*s fills the room as voices with different volumes bounce off the tan plaster walls. After about five seconds, a few voices begin dropping off, and, soon thereafter, a few more, and then, still more, everyone digging deep to find their last ounces of air to expel, all of us simultaneously opening our mouths wide to work on facial muscles that have failed or presumably will.

Eventually, I hear only George's voice.

"Ahhhhh" he continues, for several more seconds, his lungs nearly empty, fighting his disease with his breath.

"Ahhhhh. . . !"

Finally running out of air, he turns his head, first to the left, and then to the right. He then lifts his chin and flashes a cat-that-ate-the-canary smirk.

"What do you think of that?" he says.

I laugh . . . and I am hooked.

OH NO!

Around this same time, I take my daughter Meredith to her weekly piano lesson and speak with her teacher for the first time since my diagnosis. We have known Jeanine for many years and consider her a family friend. A fun, attractive, hip, and artsy musician, she embodies the joys of creativity and youthful freedom.

As she says hello, my stomach tosses a late lunch from one of its sides to the other. My heartbeat quickens. I feel clammy even though the back of my neck tingles with heat.

We hug, talk briefly, and feeling my pulse slowing down, I gently exhale. I feel good about our exchange, with what I say and how I say it. It seems natural and I even make her laugh. Not bad, I think to myself, and especially for someone with an "old person's disease."

As she and Meredith walk into the other room to begin the lesson, I look down and notice that my fly is open! Wide as can be for the whole world to see. The old man's classic burden.

I quickly zip up, walk outside, and call Tracey to tell her what occurred.

"You won't believe what just happened," I say.

When I tell her, she starts laughing. Hard. And she can't stop.

"When it rains, it pours," I say, 'but at least I didn't fart as I turned and walked away!"

"Well, there is that," she says.

Now, we are both laughing, almost crying, in fact. My aching stomach tells the story.

Before hanging up and walking to my car, where I will wait for Meredith to finish her lesson, I check my zipper one more time.

HMMM

David Foster Wallace once said, "There are forms of humor that escape pain, and there are forms of humor that transfigure pain."[1] With Parkinson's, I have discovered that trying to find humor in distressing or awkward situations helps to humanize them—that is, to remind me that they're fairly common and, typically, less worrisome than I might think. And humanizing them helps to transform them into something less dreadful, less threatening, less absurd. That is why finding and using humor remains essential as I live with the absurdity of Parkinson's.

I often say, "Sometimes we have to laugh so that we don't cry."

As George understands, and Tracey, too, what better choice do we have?

1. Wallace, "Interview."

12

SLOWING DOWN

"He was always in a hurry to get where he was not."

—Leo Tolstoy, *War and Peace*

HURRYING

Parkinson's disease affects your ability to move. It makes you stiff, impairs your balance, causes you to shake, and slows you down. In fact, *bradykinesia*, the official term for this slowing down, is a cardinal symptom of the disease.

It is the summer of 2017, about nine months since my Parkinson's diagnosis. On vacation in Surfside Beach, South Carolina, with my wife, our daughters, and my parents, I awake earlier than usual one morning. Having slept like a man without a care, I am now eager to start the day.

Faint rays of early dawn drop through the skylight above our bed without constraint, which hastens me to the coffee pot downstairs. With no one else awake, after making the coffee I decide to take a walk on the beach. We have a busy day ahead of us, so I will soon need to hustle back to our rented beach house and usher my children out of bed.

Walking barefoot, the beach sand feels cool between my toes. Dry at first, it becomes damp as I move closer to the water. Looking in both directions, I can see a couple dozen people who have beaten me there, though the beach still feels mostly untouched. Gentle humid breezes blow, and I see an older couple walking side by side on the water's edge, also barefoot and moving at a calm pace. Both of them occasionally bend down to examine washed up seashells of most every shape imaginable. The choppy ocean waters glisten behind them.

The man picks up a shell and shows it to his companion, and her face takes on the form of an "ooh" as she rubs the small of his back with her hand. Additional tender gestures between them prompt several reciprocated smiles. I wonder how long they have been together, what joys they have shared, and what heartaches they have endured.

With the tide going out, I can still see fragments of jagged shells and salty froth that mark the waterline from the previous night's high tide. The beach service that drags this debris away each morning has not yet passed by.

A lone seagull flying low in search of food caws. Drawn to it for a brief moment before looking down at my watch, I see it is time to return to the beach house, so I turn, pick up my pace, and hurry back.

We need to plan our day.

SLOWING DOWN

While walking briskly, I see someone who reminds me of a man I met a previous summer, when the four of us visited my parents just a few miles away in a town called Pawley's Island, where they lived at the time.

I flash back to this memory.

One afternoon, we make a visit to Brookgreen Gardens, a wildlife preserve and sculpture garden located nearby. On a warm, still, and humid day, after walking around the gardens for over an hour and feeling the effects of the heat, we search for a shady place to sit down. A covered pontoon boat, which, we learn, travels in the slightly cooler marshes of the Lowcountry, looks inviting.

We ask a young woman selling tickets on the makeshift dock how long the boat ride lasts. I'd made plans for us to have an early dinner.

"I think we'll have time if we hustle," I say to Tracey. She lets out a faint sigh.

The boat's captain welcomes us aboard. A man who appears to be in his fifties, with leathery tanned skin, tells some of his story, which, as we learn, has unfolded in these marshes and the nearby ocean.

We push off from the dock, and as he steers the boat slowly through calm tidal creeks lined by beautiful sweetgrass, live oaks, and saw palmetto shrubs, he waxes eloquent about life in this part of the world. A floating encyclopedia, he speaks about the region's wildlife, plant life, and customs with the conviction of a street preacher and the reverence of a cloistered monk.

Then, he cuts off the boat's trolling motor, which slows our momentum and leaves us floating calmly in the dark reedy water.

"My philosophy is to never be in a hurry," he says. "Never."

"Wherever I look, people are hurrying to get somewhere . . . anywhere . . . and why? The years pass quickly. We're on this earth for such a short time," he says.

His tone is resolute, but not judgmental.

My eyes meet Tracey's. For decades, she has told me the same thing.

"I learned as a young fella that, whether I'm driving my boat in the creeks or my pickup on the highway, when I go too fast I miss beautiful and interesting things," he says. "Things right in front of me. Things I won't see again."

Then, pointing first to a heron in flight and next to a magnolia tree in bloom, he grins and says, "You miss a lot when you're in a hurry."

BREATHING

I slow my pace and turn toward the small waves barely breaking on the beach, stopping at the water's edge. Looking out over the choppy ocean, I see an enormous bare horizon. A gentle breeze blows as a young child, walking alongside her mother, squeals. Several seagulls circle overhead, and moments later a large school of fish darkens the water as it passes by.

An unusually shaped shell catches my eye, popping with various colors before the white froth washes over it.

Slowly breathing in the salt air, I press my bare feet into the cool wet sand, wishing that Tracey and the girls were with me.

13

MISDIAGNOSED

———

Parkinson's disease can be difficult to diagnose, even for seasoned physicians. A main reason is that, particularly in its early stages, Parkinson's shares numerous symptoms with other illnesses.[1] As a result, having a neurologist trained in movement disorders, or what we call a movement disorder specialist (MDS), is vitally important, not only for treatment but also for diagnosis.

Up to 35 percent of those living with Parkinson's disease, or one in three, tell stories of an initial misdiagnosis.[2]

I'll share my story.

WORRYING

Dr. W walks into the exam room. She has been my doctor since we moved to Austin in 2003. In fact, she is my wife, Tracey's, doctor, too, and we both adore her. She has an ideal mix of traits for a physician: smart, relational, patient, and funny. In her fifties, and with fair skin, light freckles, short brown curly hair, and glasses, she has a kind, inviting smile even when resting her face. Long legs and a thin build reveal that she is a runner, as

———

1. "Conditions that Mimic Parkinson's."

2. Schrag, Ben-Shlomo, and Quinn, "How Valid is the Clinical Diagnosis of Parkinson's Disease in the Community?"

does the thick black band of her watch. Her specialty in sports and family medicine suits her well.

"I'm here because I need you to tell me I'm not dying," I say.

"We're *all* dying," she says.

I laugh. She flashes her now big, kind smile.

"So, you have a twitchy finger?" she says.

Having experienced a faint tremor in my left index finger for a few weeks, I told her nurse about it before Dr. W arrived.

I lift up my finger, point at the wall, and it begins to twitch. She moves closer to the exam table, where I sit.

"Well, at the very least, I need you to tell me I don't have Parkinson's or ALS," I say.

Her face takes on a more pensive expression. Her tone becomes more measured.

"Let's see what's going on," she says.

I begin to feel hot inside and the back of my neck tingles.

Turning around, she takes her handheld light from the small counter beside the exam table, which also holds a box of tongue depressors, gauze, latex gloves, and other supplies.

Looking into each of my eyes, she asks me to follow her fingers as she moves them to different places. She then asks me to stick out my tongue and hold it, like my daughters used to do when mad at each other. Born twenty-three months apart, they still fuss at one another sometimes, but they also say "I love you" and they give each other hugs before going to bed.

Next, Dr. W asks me to move my tongue back and forth inside my mouth, from cheek to cheek. I follow each of her commands dutifully.

Finally, she has me roll my arms, one over the other, as if I am playing patty cake with a young child. After I do this several times, and in alternating directions, her expression becomes even more serious. Hot waves begin to move through my body.

"Allan, I'm sorry, but I can't tell you that you don't have Parkinson's or ALS," she says.

"What?" I whisper. "What do you mean? What concerns you? The finger tremor?"

"I'm more concerned about your left arm. It's stiff, almost locked up; and it's more noticeable when you roll it over the other arm, in both directions."

Silence.

I swallow hard. I'm forty-eight years old with two young children.

"Are you more concerned about Parkinson's or ALS?" I ask.

"Parkinson's . . . but let's not get ahead of ourselves. It would be unusual for a person your age to have it. But if you do have it, it's early, and it's slow-progressing, and it's treatable for a long time. Many years."

I volunteer to do the exercise again. I will just keep trying until I get it right.

"I want you to go get a massage. Let's see if we can loosen you up. If it's not better in a couple of weeks, we will go from there," she says.

I've read about Parkinson's after it came up in my Google searches, which I began in earnest after noticing my twitchy finger. I know how rare it would be for a person my age and with no family history to have it.

Still, *she* is worried about it.

She breaks the silence.

"It's *my* job to worry . . . I would like you to go ahead and schedule an appointment with Dr. T. He is a neurologist, and an expert on Parkinson's. It will likely take a few weeks to get in to see him. By that time, we should know whether your stiffness is getting better," she says.

I nod slowly in agreement, trying to push away the walls closing in on me.

"I want to know how you're doing in a couple of weeks. But remember, it's *my* job to worry," she tells me again.

REELING

I leave her office, and instead of driving back to campus, I go home. As I give Tracey the quick version of what Dr. W has just said, and tell her that she wants me to schedule an appointment with Dr. T, I dial the number to his office.

"I'm sure she just wants to be thorough," Tracey says. "You know she's like that. That's good."

I force myself to agree, but think: *You, of all people, aren't worried?* You must be in denial, because you always worry about health stuff.

The receptionist tells me that the first available appointment is nearly a month away, but I take it.

"Please call me if you have a cancellation. Any appointment time is fine. I'll make it work," I say.

As I hang up, Tracey comes into the bedroom. Her salt-and-pepper hair is pulled back from her face, and the long sleeves of her autumn orange cotton T-shirt are pushed up because she's been baking. A few specks of white flour rest on her high olive cheekbone.

"What all did Dr. W say?" she asks.

I share more details of the exam, and tell her about the need for a massage.

Tracey restates her thorough approach to care.

I interrupt her.

"It's going to be almost a month before I can see the neurologist," I say, "and I can't wait that long. I will lose my mind . . . I'm going to call David."

I send a text to my friend, who is a physician in Austin.

Can you give me a call when you have a moment?

He calls almost immediately, and I tell him what's going on and ask if he can help me get in to see another neurologist.

"I'd like to see someone as quickly as possible," I say.

"I understand . . . Let me speak with some colleagues and I'll give you a call back," he says.

I thank him, hang up, and pace the house.

A few minutes later, he calls back and gives me the name of a neurologist, Dr. R, whom a colleague has suggested.

"I don't know her, but another doctor says she's good. She and I just spoke, and she is expecting you to call . . . I don't know about her experience with Parkinson's, but maybe she can be helpful. It's a start," he says.

I thank him.

"Let me know how it goes. I'll keep working on other possibilities," he says.

We hang up and I call Dr. R's office.

"This is Allan Cole. My friend, Dr. David Navale, suggested I call. I've been referred to a neurologist . . . tremor in my index finger . . . stiffness in my arm . . .earliest available, please."

"Hold on a moment, please."

I wait.

"Mr. Cole, she can see you at 4 PM today, if that works."

"Wonderful. Thank you so much. I'll see you then," I say.

I head to my office, trying to get my mind on something else. I have four hours to wait.

HOPING

"You have a physiologic tremor," she says, after giving me a thorough examination. "It's nothing to worry about."

I exhale like a whale rising to the ocean's surface.

Dr. R's calm face matches her reassuring tone. Her dark wire-rimmed glasses enhance her already apparent intellect and give me extra confidence in what she is saying.

"Let me show you," she says, gesturing for me to take a seat and pointing to her laptop screen. I read it.

Physiologic tremor . . .occurs in healthy individuals . . . not considered a disease, but is a normal phenomenon . . . enhanced by stress and anxiety . . . .

"See, nothing to worry about," she says.

Butterflies rush out of my stomach.

"Thank you. I'm *so* relieved, and I can't tell you how much I appreciate your kindness and generosity. Getting me in so quickly made such a difference," I say.

I almost reach out to hug her, but catch myself.

"I'm happy to deliver good news," she says.

I stand up, shake her hand, and walk to the checkout desk to give the receptionist my co-pay.

Looking at the paperwork, she says, "No follow-up appointment is needed."

I smile like a kid on his birthday.

Walking to my car, I text Tracey.

I'm fine. A benign tremor.

Thank God. I'm relieved, she writes.

Me too. I'll call later.

I love you, honey, she writes, adding several heart emojis.

I smile, and remember the few months after we met, when she was finishing college in New York and I, having just graduated, lived in North Carolina. We talked daily on the telephone, back when doing that cost a lot of money, and we sent each other cards and faxes with sappy notes that young loves find thrilling. We still leave each other sappy notes, and, in recent years, lots of emojis. It is still thrilling.

I head back to my office to finish a couple of things. The fall semester has just begun and it is a typically full week.

DOUBTING

At dinner that evening, we gather around our kitchen's island and talk about the day. Holly, our third grader, tells us about her upcoming math test, and that she is learning her multiplication tables. She begins to recite them and gets up to six times six, before being distracted by our dog Sunny, who's in our fenced front yard and, as usual, barks at someone walking by.

Meredith, our fifth grader, begins telling us about a kid at school who told her that boys think farts are funnier than girls do, and that she told him he's being sexist.

Holly walks outside to play with Sunny, and Meredith heads to her room with the iPad.

"In ten minutes, you have to finish your homework," I tell her.

"You got it, Daddo," she says, already mesmerized by her screen.

"I'm so happy you got a good report today," Tracey says.

"Me too," I say.

"I know you were worried," she says, "and I was, too . . . but I figured there's no way you could have Parkinson's disease. It didn't add up."

"Maybe not," I say, "But I'm keeping my appointment with Dr. T . . . ."

14

LOSING YOUR DOCTOR

RECEIVING NOTICE

The letter arrives about two years after that fateful morning, when I was only forty-eight and he uttered those life-changing words, "I think you're in the beginning stages of Parkinson's disease."

I should have anticipated the letter. After all, at my second appointment he said he expected to practice "another couple of years." Not only this, but looking back he had already reduced his hours and worked three days a week. Perhaps he wanted to wean me, and hundreds of others, off his life-sustaining care. Maybe he hoped to wean himself after four plus decades of a dedicated professional life.

Either way, he said, "When the time comes, I'll make sure you get with another neurologist who will take good care of you."

I knew all along that the time would come too soon.

"It's been a privilege taking care of you . . . ," the letter says, and a lump forms in my throat and emptiness numbs my chest, like when moving away from my best friends in middle school or when a former girlfriend told me that she wanted to break up. Now that I am age fifty-one, the adult world's norms do not temper my despair.

A UNIQUE LOSS

Why might losing a doctor prompt such primitive and painful emotions?

It must have something to do with vulnerability.

In the medical relationship, from start to finish, patients dwell in a vulnerable place. Always exposed and often compromised, whether physically, emotionally, or both, we yield power over our bodies and futures while simultaneously pledging deep trust and forming our greatest hopes.

Our doctors have hopes for us, too, and for relieving our plight. It can be difficult to detect this hope. Many doctors *and* patients assume that the professional relationship prescribes impermeable boundaries. At their worst, these boundaries can place great emotional distance between us, and can inform what philosopher Michel Foucault termed "the medical gaze," wherein the doctor focuses on the body as separate from the person's larger identity.[1] Even so, in most cases, I believe, a measure of shared hope marks this unique relationship.

Of course, we enter into this relationship willingly and with trust because the stakes of being, staying, or getting healthy remain high. For those of us with acute or chronic illnesses, any relationship with a doctor begins and evolves with us in need. We need to feel better, to reduce symptoms, to build strength, and, as much as any of this, to have good quality of life. Therefore, we place great hope in our doctor's ability to treat us and to care for us; and with each visit, as our shared history builds, our shared hope can build, too.

Importantly, we place our hope not merely in a person, the doctor, but even more so in the relationship, imbalanced though it may have to be. Our hope remains tethered to experiences of care marked by empathy, listening, consultation, and collaboration.

Maybe, then, losing a doctor makes us lose hope.

MOURNING AND REINVESTING

Obviously, we cannot prevent losing a doctor. Besides, doctors have the right to retire as much as anyone else does. But our doctor retiring, or closing a practice, or, as I also experienced, dying, differs from when any of this happens with our barber, dentist, or accountant, as important as these relationships may be. Losing our doctor, who knows us in such detail, so

---

1. Foucault, *The Birth of the Clinic.*

intimately, and to whose care we entrust our lives, can feel like its own kind of death.

As a result, recognizing this unique type of loss, and mourning it, are both necessary and appropriate, even as we reinvest by seeking out a new doctor with whom to be vulnerable, to develop trust, and to rebuild hope.

It's my last appointment with my doctor nearing retirement, and after leaving the exam room and walking together toward the front desk, we stop and I extend my hand.

"I'll always be grateful for you," I say. "I'm happy for you . . . and I'll miss you."

The lump in my throat returns. So does the emptiness in my chest.

"You're going to do well . . . and it's been my pleasure," he says.

I want to say more, but I don't.

Slowly leaving his office, I take the elevator to the parking garage and get in my car.

I wipe my eyes before driving to work.

15

THE IMPORTANCE OF BEGINNINGS

"The beginning in every task is the chief thing."

—Plato

RUNNING

Somewhere near the small central Texas town of Wallis, I am running my second of three legs in the Texas Independence Relay. It is after 3 AM on a Sunday morning and I have not slept in twenty-two hours.

I am on a team of twelve runners. Five of us have Parkinson's disease but it touches us all. Our team captain and my new friend, Craig Potts, lives with Parkinson's and has brought us all together. It will take us nearly thirty-six hours to complete the 200-mile route, which ends in Houston. Having begun the previous morning in the town of Gonzales, we are over halfway there.

Navigating a rough dirt road, I find a good running cadence under a clear, starlit sky. The world is warm, still, and quiet. I hear only my feet hitting the road and the air moving rhythmically in and out of my lungs. The LED headlamp strapped over my Houston Astros baseball cap shines a few feet in front of me, illuminating the tranquil dark sky. If I turn my head slightly to the right or left, I glimpse a swath of massive bluebonnet fields that surround me.

It is March of 2018, nearly eighteen months since learning I have Parkinson's. Still tinged with anxiety much of the time, my thoughts linger this early morning on lessons I am learning, about myself and others; lessons on illness and resilience, on darkness and light.

LEARNING

I am learning the importance of getting to know other people who have Parkinson's disease, something I could not do for nearly a year after my diagnosis, when I lived in the Parkinson's closet. Even after publicly sharing my diagnosis, before becoming friends with Craig I knew little more than a handful of people who have the disease. Now, as I get to know my other teammates who live with Parkinson's—Allie, Bob, Deanna, and Alex, our videographer—I have a sense of calm that has been so elusive. These new relationships put me at ease and make my experience feel more normal. Our conversations spark inspiration and new wisdom. Spending time with my Parkinson's kin offers a previously unimagined feeling of hope, one tethered to being in solidarity. To my surprise, I am learning how close you can feel to another person you have only just met, simply because you both have the same insidious disease.

It's a beginning.

I am also learning the healing power of living with openness and vulnerability, especially when tied to a measure of authenticity you never thought possible. We wear masks, after all, and more often than we realize. They conceal our pain, but precisely because they prevent its expression these masks can intensify it and allow it to have an even more destructive influence.

Of course, there are many people in the world of whom we should never ask for more vulnerability: those who are poor, abused, neglected, marginalized, or victimized. But many of us have much to gain by removing our mask, at least for a bit, and allowing others to glimpse our humanity in its more exposed and unvarnished forms.

Kierkegaard asked, "Are you not aware that there comes a midnight hour when everyone must unmask?"[1] If nothing else, I am learning from Parkinson's the benefits of unmasking earlier than the midnight hour. These benefits include a sense of calm, healing, and hope.

Another beginning.

1. Kierkegaard, *Either/Or*, Part II, 146.

Parkinson's will never define me, but it certainly guides me. Like an LED headlamp, it illumines paths in front of me: those of illness and health, scarcity and abundance, suffering and joy, mystery and understanding. It also gets me outside of myself and points me toward *others*, and this invites me to put Parkinson's to work on behalf of something life-giving. In this respect, I am learning the importance of embodying *compassion*—which literally means "to suffer with"—and joining with others to alleviate suffering. Trying to help ease another person's pain or burden helps to lessen my own, and all of us who travel the Parkinson's road, or one like it, are sturdier, more resilient, and more hopeful *together*.

Still another beginning.

LIVING

After lifting up the front of my Team Fox shirt to wipe sweat from my eyes, I begin to run faster. With the next relay transfer point less than a mile ahead, the support van that has been checking on me honks and goes by one last time, carrying half of my teammates. The other half, already in town, await our arrival.

Running another hundred yards and making a right turn, I see the uneven dirt road change to smooth, flat pavement. Ahead of me, the yellow glow from several old fashioned street lamps hangs in the air.

I shift into an even higher gear and feel like I'm gliding.

My breathing quickens. Radiant stars, as numerous as the bluebonnets at my feet, reach from the night sky and hold my gaze. I hark back to something I read years before, when I was graduate student studying the work of Erik H. Erikson, a twentieth-century psychologist. I had forgotten if I ever really believed it.

Erikson's wife and collaborator, Joan Erickson, observed that regardless of our age, from cradle to grave, "Life doesn't make any sense without interdependence. We need each other, and the sooner we learn that, the better for us all."[2]

I keep running toward the yellow glow, toward my team.

The road straightens, and beneath a row of lights that line one side of the downtown street stands a thickening crowd of people, mostly other runners, all of them cheering; all a part of something bigger than themselves. I see my teammates: Allie, Bob, Emily, Deanna, Ron, Kristi, Shae, Amy, and

2. Goleman, "Erickson, in His Own Old Age."

Salvador. Some wave their arms, others clap, another rings a cowbell, their collective cheers growing louder as I pass by.

High-fiving Craig, I pump my arms and start the final kick toward the transfer point a couple of hundred yards away, where I'll pass the baton to Lori and our collective cheers will land on her.

My thoughts drift again: to my wife, to our daughters, to my mom and dad, to trusted friends and colleagues, to my Parkinson's kin, to the better way I am beginning to live.

And beginnings matter.

16

TALKING MYSELF INTO HOPE

HURTING

As the midday sun shines through our bedroom window, a few specks of dust dance through the air. I turn on the rustic coffee-brown ceiling fan that hangs over our bed and the dust immediately vanishes.

My wife is out running errands with our daughters. The three of them baked peanut butter and M&M cookies before leaving the house and a wonderfully warm smell lingers in every room.

I sit down on the bed, and the deep blues in our comforter and pillow shams offer me momentary calm. My eyes wander to Meredith's colorful cubist self-portrait hanging on the wall next to my side of the bed. Then I turn to Holly's simple black silhouette, which hangs on the adjacent wall, closer to the end of the bed. I smile, rubbing my hand back and forth across the soft comforter before lying back on the mattress.

Staring at the ceiling fan as it slowly spins, I take off on the roller coaster I have come to call "the Low Dopamine Express," which has become all too familiar in the last few months. I climb slowly up Apathy Hill, flatten out for a moment before speeding down Sadness Drop, and then, at top speed, I spring quickly sideways into the long pull toward Anxiety Alley before slowing down, turning again, and starting the upward climb once more.

Six months have passed since my Parkinson's diagnosis. Plagued by questions, darkness hovers and hope evades me.

TALKING TO MYSELF

Almost immediately after my diagnosis, at the urging of a massage thera-pist, I began a brief stretching routine before getting out of bed each morn-ing. It relieves muscle stiffness, helps me focus, and provides a good start to the day.

One morning, as I lie in bed and stretch my hands, wrists, and fore-arms, but before moving to leg, ankle, and foot stretches, I say these words:

I am grateful for another day.
I will do my best to make it good.
I will focus on my strengths.
I will be hopeful.

I say the words aloud, several times, so that I hear myself speak them. I repeat them the next morning, too, and the next. Soon thereafter, I begin saying them not only in the morning but several times throughout the day, and especially when I start to worry, feel afraid, or otherwise despair.

I am grateful for another day.
I will do my best to make it good.
I will focus on my strengths.
I will be hopeful.

Over time, and with practice, I notice changes in how I think about my life with Parkinson's, how I feel about the challenges it presents, and even how I mourn the losses I've already experienced as well as those I anticipate.

I've begun talking myself into hope.

I know this, not because the pain of loss, fear, and uncertainty goes away, but because I have begun to see things differently.

HOPING

One new way of seeing things comes to me in a dream.

I see a tree. Tall, thick trunked, and sturdy, its broad canopy reaches dozens of feet across the sky and provides generous shade in every direc-tion. Similar to a large red cedar in my front yard, this tree in my dream stands alone, independent, its green leafy cover having long pushed out any close presence of other trees. Appearing confident and robust, it conveys protection, safety, and support for life.

Then, I notice a field of bright yellow wildflowers. They cover the landscape as far as I can see. As a gentle wind blows, this floral blanket takes on different contours, its colorful blooms swaying back and forth. They twist and turn through the countryside in solidarity, petal to petal, stem to stem, displaying resilience and radiating beauty, regardless of the wind's strength or direction.

As I take in their splendor, I see a different kind of strength. It's forged from togetherness, freedom, and the resolve to be what they are. Nothing more.

I often conjure up their memory.

Especially when talking myself into hope.

17

A MAN AT THE LAKE

I see him just after sunrise most Sunday mornings, when I run at the lake. Partially covered by a frayed and faded gray bandana, his long salt-and-pepper dreadlocks hang down over his thick shoulders and muscular frame. Beside him on the ground lay his few belongings, which fit neatly into two large duffel bags fastened to a folding steel utility cart.

Holding a makeshift walking stick, he often stands at the water's edge and stares across the lake; at times quietly, sometimes speaking, occasionally chanting with rhythmic intonations.

Each morning when I run on the north side of the lake, I anticipate seeing this man and wonder what he will be doing. I have seen him shout in frustration, shaking his fist while he looks to the sky. I have watched him plead in desperation with his opened hands in front of his face. I have even seen him on his knees in a posture of reverence, his head bowed and hands clasped, and heard his tone of peaceful resolve.

Whatever his mood or posture, he says his truth over the waters.

We have never spoken, but I imagine him being there to cast out his demons, those tied to poverty, homelessness, mental illness, and perhaps other difficulties. I might have it all wrong, of course; it's presumptuous of me to imagine in this way. But something about the waters draws him there, day after day, week after week, year after year.

Is it their serenity, beauty, or power to birth and sustain life? Is it their qualities of renewal, or ability to help bracket daily struggles, leaving us feeling more grounded and whole?

On any given day, hundreds of other runners, walkers, and cyclists pass by him as they traverse the ten-mile trail that wraps around the lake. A few people offer a half glance in his direction. Some catch him peripherally and quicken their pace. Most seem unfazed. Perhaps their own demons, or those of loved ones, consume them.

Parkinson's disease can itself feel demonic, and precisely because it proves so consuming. It grabs and takes hold of you and over time requires more of your attention and energy while simultaneously draining it away.

As Parkinson's progresses, it may also bring additional symptoms that need managing—muscle cramping (dystonia), tremors, gait or balance problems, swallowing difficulties, sleep disturbance, constipation, and more. Progression usually requires taking more medicine. With this medicine come side effects, as well as extra trips to the drug store and added visits to multiple care providers: movement disorder specialists, physical therapists, and speech therapists. This cascade of events can prompt consuming anxiety or depression—or both—which creates a need for adding still more care team members, more medicine, and yet more therapeutic support.

Having Parkinson's is a full-time gig, day after day, week after week, year after year.

Which brings me back to the man at the lake. At first blush, he and I have so little in common; me so privileged and resourced, he presumably poor, homeless, mentally ill, and living at the margins. But I believe we both live with demons tethered to chronic illness, and we both try to limit their power, their all-consuming grip, in our journeys to the waters, he by speaking, me by running; and I wonder if, like me, his presence there gives him a sense of freedom that comes with feeling fully alive.

Either way, I am drawn to him; I am drawn to his shouting, his pleading, his bowing at the water's edge.

You might be, too.

18

POWER IN ACCEPTANCE

HIDING

One afternoon, just before two o'clock, I watch him enter the main conference room in the College of Pharmacy. My enviably handsome and bright colleague, an accomplished neurologist, arrives with a couple of other colleagues. He walks toward me as the other two take seats on the far side of the large square table. A few others will soon trickle in.

Twelve of us, all senior-level administrators from The University of Texas's schools of medicine, pharmacy, nursing, and social work, meet several times each year to discuss how best to collaborate in interprofessional education. Our shared goal is to prepare our students—future doctors, nurses, pharmacists, and social workers—to work together on professional teams in the complex world of health care. This is the first time we have all met since my diagnosis, and none of my colleagues knows I have Parkinson's.

Other than our friends, Stacey and Paul, my friend, Dana Bliss, who is also my editor at Oxford University Press, and my doctors, no one else knows.

Placing his phone and small notebook on the table, my colleague sits down beside me while I try to find the sweet spot in an uncomfortable chair. We greet each other and exchange pleasantries, as we have done many times before, and then engage in small talk while waiting for the rest of our group to arrive.

As he speaks, my stomach tosses what I have eaten for lunch from one of its sides to the other, and my heart beats faster. I feel clammy and it becomes harder to breathe as my internal monologue begins.

Can he tell I have Parkinson's?

Is his smile one of pity?

Does he think I'm less effective in my job?

Will he say something to my boss?

I'll bet he's writing me off as a colleague, already taking me less seriously.

His work focuses on strokes, but he must know about my condition. As an accomplished neurologist, he can probably spot Parkinson's a mile away.

I'm so sorry you've got it, but your secret is safe with me, I imagine him thinking as he remains cordial and keeps talking.

The rest of our colleagues arrive and the meeting begins, but I have little recollection of it. For nearly two hours, choppy waves roll through my body. At times, the room blurs and its walls encroach. Hearing the conversation, but not absorbing anything, I remain silent. Pretending to take notes and occasionally nodding in agreement, I hope I can keep playing along. *Willing* myself into participating, while tucking my twitchy left index finger under my leg, becomes the goal. The hands on a large wall clock inch forward and could not care less.

Just before the meeting ends, my neurologist colleague takes a phone call and leaves the room. My pulse slows and my breathing relaxes. The room begins to feel bigger. One colleague speaks about steps before our next meeting. I look at the calendar on my phone and begin counting the days.

RISKING

Nearly three years later, I am out of the Parkinson's closet, managing my disease, living my life, and, yes, doing my job. Nothing has changed professionally, although having a progressive disease means acknowledging that change always looms. What has changed is that I recognize what was happening at that meeting. I now understand better the roots of my paralyzing fear. The threat of losing your identity as a healthy person, and soon thereafter losing your professional standing, can be disorienting. Assuming that others would see me as ill and as "less than" I was before was, I recoiled at the prospect of their pity and dismissal.

Now, I recognize something more. Because I feared perceiving *myself* in these ways, I attributed the same perceptions to *others*. Whether having to do with illness or with most any other life experience, we tend to make assumptions about what other people think and feel, about all kinds of matters but especially about ourselves. Frequently these prove merely to be our own assumptions and self-perceptions. In psychological terms, we call this a *projection*.

A fear of losing our identity and status is legitimate. Choosing to live openly with any chronic condition comes with risk, social and professional. Whether subtle or overt, discrimination may occur. Moreover, a fear of losing key parts of ourselves jars us from comforts we grow accustomed to and, perhaps, take for granted. I am thinking of the comforts of the familiar and of feeling accepted among our most cherished groups of people and in our most coveted spaces.

Maya Angelou recognized this common human need to feel accepted, observing that, "The ache for home lives in all of us. The safe place where we can go as we are and not be questioned."[1] I am learning that having a chronic illness spurs my aching for home precisely because it disrupts my safe places. But it also shows me that these safe places may be found where I am already—among family, friends, neighbors, and colleagues, most of whom accept and even root for me—and that my foremost challenge may be to accept and root for myself.

1. Angelou, *All God's Children Need Traveling Shoes,* 196.

19

BROOKLYN, CENTRAL PARK, AND THE BIRD

CHILLS

Certain things about that extraordinary day three years ago remain stamped in my memory, when Tracey, my partner of twenty-seven years, ran the New York City Marathon and I was there with our daughters, cheering for her.

There was the bright blue sky that covered the city that pristine fall day; and Tracey running up 4th Avenue in Brooklyn dressed in purple New Balance shoes with a matching shirt and headband; and her face radiating joyful freedom and fierce determination. I also remember our girls holding a sign they had made that read, "Go Mom! Bib #29292"; and I can still picture Tracey wrapped in a royal blue warming poncho that she received when crossing the finish line in Central Park, the look on her face now showing equal parts exhaustion and elation.

These memories continue to captivate me.

They always will.

But there are also gaps in my memory. Only eleven days earlier, my doctor delivered the bone-chilling news that I had Parkinson's disease at the age of forty-eight. As is true for many people, I was riding along a smooth road in midlife—raising young children, enjoying a successful career, making plans for the future—and I got T-boned at an intersection I never saw. I had to acknowledge losing an imaginary control over my life. More than that, I feared my life was over.

INSIGHTS

When I return to New York in a couple of weeks to run my own marathon, I expect to form new and less gap-filled memories. Now inhabiting a different emotional space, I know that I can live a full life with this illness, and that as changes occur and challenges present themselves I can adapt, compensate, and, when needed, simply accept a new normal and reset my expectations for this full life. Adjusting your expectations goes a long way when seeking meaning, endurance, and peace with chronic illness. This I have learned from cohabitating with the Parkinson's beast.

I have learned other things. One is that medicine is at once miraculous and maddening, able to treat many illnesses, including Parkinson's, but not necessarily able to cure them. This reality requires setting expectations accordingly, hoping for better treatments and a cure, believing they will come because the science says so, while recognizing that progressive diseases progress and that to *live* means not betting it all on the future but also cashing in today.

I have learned, too, that children are typically better at talking about hard things than we assume, are usually better at it than grown-ups, and that a child's honesty, courage, and resilience can inspire our own. As excruciating as sharing bad news with your children can be, it can turn out to be good, for them and for you.

Keeping secrets can destroy you.

Tracey, Meredith, Holly and I speak openly and honestly about my Parkinson's. We pose and answer questions, talk about new drugs and therapies being developed, celebrate friends doing good work to raise awareness and funds for research, try to make our own contributions, and we can even be playful about it all. Still, we only talk about Parkinson's issues when there is the need. More often, we talk about theater and dance, school and friends, sleepovers and swim parties, our dogs and pet bird, our hopes and dreams.

I have also learned anew that there is a lot of suffering around us, *all the time*, and that we can begin to notice its contours and textures more readily when we ourselves suffer. As Tracey always says, "Everyone has their shit." Because I know Tracey is right, I find enormous value in living openly with my illness, which includes speaking honestly about it when others mention it or when it feels appropriate for me to discuss it. Putting others at ease with my illness helps me feel more at ease, and talking about Parkinson's helps educate people and can lead to their involvement with finding cures and offering support. Furthermore, transparency with my disease can also invite others to share their own struggles, fears, and needs with me, which allows me to support them and deepens our relationship.

I never imagined that having Parkinson's would teach me any of this, and so much more.

WARMTH

Back to the marathon. I have run it numerous times in my imagination, visualizing what it will be like to join 50,000 runners, including several of my Team Fox friends, and wind through the five boroughs of New York.

Several people have asked about my race goals. My goals are modest, really. I hope to enjoy myself, to soak in the energy of it all, but most of all to hug my family and friends along the route and tell them I love them, celebrate them, and remain grateful for their support. I suspect they will see my face reflecting a deep sense of freedom and determination, exhaustion and elation. If my good fortune continues, I will also wrap a warming poncho around myself at the finish line with an overflowing heart.

Then, walking through Central Park and thinking of my many sisters and brothers who live with this cruel disease, I'll flip Parkinson's the bird.

With both hands.

20

UNFINISHED SPACES
AND SPIRITUAL THINGS

UNFINISHED SPACES

"Over there is the Cathedral of St. John the Divine," I say. Peering out the large windows of our rented apartment and pointing across 110th Street, I gesture to my wife and our daughters, "Come take a look."

It is a Friday afternoon in early November and we have just arrived in New York for a long weekend. Three years have passed since my Parkinson's diagnosis, almost to the day. Sunday I will run the New York City Marathon.

Located a few blocks from Columbia University, this cathedral remains unfinished even though its construction began in the late nineteenth century. As a graduate student at Columbia in the 1990s, I occasionally went to St. John's to find solitude and to reflect on life's bigger questions: those of meaning, purpose, and hope.

Scaffolding and work crews notwithstanding, the cathedral has a long, beautiful, Gothic-style nave that still captivates me. This sanctuary—a place of refuge—draws visitors of every nation and creed. It attracts people from a variety of religious and spiritual traditions as well as those living with more questions than answers. Seekers and skeptics, themselves unfinished and on paths of discovery, journey to this place. I suspect that, like me, many who visit long to gain more insight, perhaps to unload their burdens, and even to catch a glimpse of the divine.

Tracey and I will take our girls there on Monday, the day after the marathon.

SPIRITUAL THINGS

It's the evening before the marathon that grips me now, when I experienced another kind of sanctuary.

Those of us running for Team Fox—120 in total and four of us with Parkinson's—gather at a Midtown restaurant for an early dinner with our families. Michael J. Fox, who has lived courageously with Parkinson's for nearly thirty years, joins us. He speaks eloquently in both humorous and poignant ways about what the Team Fox community has meant to him over the years.

Visibly moved as he looks around the room at all of us, he says, "You should see how beautiful you are," and then shares a few memories from marathons he's witnessed and speaks with joy about his foundation putting a team together each year to run.

Many of us watch with our own full heart and moist eyes.

At one point, he pauses and says, "I've been thinking about spiritual things."

He tells us that his youngest daughter's birthday sometimes falls on the day of the marathon, as it will this year, and that she was born in 2001, not long after the horrific events of 9/11. After weeks of uncertainty about there being a marathon that year, in a city carrying so much pain and with many burdens to shed, he recalls standing at his apartment window with his newborn daughter in his arms and watching crowds of marathon runners as they passed by.

He says, "I remember looking out at the people and I thought to myself ... this is beautiful; this is what people can do and how they can overcome."

Again, he pauses. Then, acknowledging that we all have our own personal pain and burdens to endure, whether because we live with Parkinson's or we love someone who does, he says, "It's the same looking out that window to look out at all of you. It means so much. I love you all. I know you are all here for your own reasons and for your own people. But we are all *our* people."

JOURNEYS

As with any chronic illness, Parkinson's makes us journeyers. Against our will, it grabs us, disorients us, and places us on a path of discovery. There we must find our bearings and search for ways to live a full life with a disease that seeks constantly to take life away.

Like those making visits to the cathedral, we who journey with this insidious disease represent every nation, creed, and spiritual path. We also live in unfinished spaces laced with profound questions of meaning, and purpose, and hope.

What's more, we have burdens to unload. We long to find healing. Often in need of maintenance if not repair, we require permanent scaffolding for support. For all of these reasons, and more, we need *all* our people.

I see this more vividly now.

In these unfinished spaces, with our people, I catch a glimpse of the divine.

21

A MORE AUTHENTIC LOVE

LOSS

Sixteen words changed my life. Spoken in one sentence on October 26, 2016, these words came from the mouth of a man I had only just met.

I was sitting in Dr. T's exam room at St. David's Medical Center in Austin, Texas. Located less than a mile from where I live, it is about halfway between my home and The University of Texas at Austin, where I work as a professor and academic dean in the Steve Hicks School of Social Work. This professional work frequently places me in positions of power, influence, and control. I am often the expert in the room, the one seated in the helping chair, and not the one awash with anxiety attached to feeling so exposed and vulnerable.

Dr. T was sitting at a small desk, focusing on me in his intent, serious way. I would come to know this look well, but at the time I was frantically searching his face, trying to predict what he was about to say before he said it.

A part of me already knew. After all, my primary care doctor had referred me to him a month earlier, and I had filled the time since with Google searches and intensive reading on medical websites. My symptoms were clear enough once I started paying attention to them.

But another part of me, the bigger part, would not allow myself even to guess what he might say. I was only forty-eight years old and had always been healthy. I had two young daughters to raise with my loving wife.

Together, we had found the sweet spot in my career, we had a bright future, we were making lots of exciting plans . . . and then he said it.

"What worries me is that I think you are in the early stages of Parkinson's disease."

DISEASE

More precisely, as I would learn, I had young-onset Parkinson's, a diagnosis given to those under the age of fifty.

A progressive neurologic disease, Parkinson's involves the loss of dopamine, a neurotransmitter in the brain that mainly affects the body's capacity for movement but also the ability to regulate one's mood, which may result in anxiety, depression, or sleep disturbance. About half of people with Parkinson's experience depression and around 40 percent will have anxiety. By the time symptoms first appear, 50 to 80 percent of a person's normal dopamine supply has already been lost, which means the disease process begins many years, even decades, before you know you have it. Though not a fatal disease per se, Parkinson's gets worse over the course of many years and typically leads to some degree of disability.

A GOOD LIFE

Before my Parkinson's diagnosis, I had always been a picture of good health. I ate well, got plenty of sleep, drank alcohol moderately, and rarely missed a day of vigorous exercise. The most serious illness I had faced was the flu. Sensitive and hopeful by nature, I also cared deeply about inequity, injustice, and people who struggled—those living on the margins of health, power, status, or hope. For over a decade I taught seminary courses and, more recently, social work courses about these and other personal and social ills, aware of my privilege and good fortune; and I wrote articles and books, too, hoping to be a voice of constructive change.

I also enjoyed the blessings of family: my wife of twenty-seven years and our two daughters. The girls were ten and eight when I received the diagnosis and I had always lived with deep gratitude for the gift of parenting them.

Before Parkinson's, life was *good*.

Surprising to me is that, three years later, I still describe myself, and my life, in these ways. Parkinson's has not changed or taken any of it.

But the disease *has* changed me.

Before Parkinson's I was fiercely private and independent. I lacked a willingness to access my deeper and more authentic emotional life, and I barred others' access, too. I rarely opened up about my feelings or my needs, even with those I cared for most: Tracey, my parents, and my closest friends. Like many people, when facing personal challenges I put my head down and plowed through them. I kept my nose to the grindstone, bit the bullet, sucked it up; and usually I did so alone. It had always been this way.

I was not a "tough guy." Nor did I embrace a hypermasculine bravado. In fact, I rejected these qualities. I taught courses and wrote books on the social constructions of gender and urged students and readers to consider and even try on broader understandings, including "masculinities." Still, I found it difficult—or more accurately, excruciatingly uncomfortable—to admit my needs, share them, or to lean on other people for support.

It was as though being vulnerable equated to weakness, as if disclosure meant becoming an object of pity or suffering a loss of respect.

As a graduate student, I came under the spell of Ralph Waldo Emerson, a nineteenth-century champion of individualism who said, "The great man is he who in the midst of the crowd keeps with perfect sweetness the independence of solitude."[1] In large part, I have lived my life accordingly.

I always hoped to become a great man.

For several months after my diagnosis, I suffered in silence, but this ultimately added to the severity of my pain because I felt so alone. The image of being stuck in the middle of a road, and knowing that a bus is coming but not exactly when, weighed on me. A lot. After nearly a half century of enviable health and youthfulness, I now had an old person's disease in middle age. I was paralyzed when thinking about the future, painfully self-conscious about my physical appearance, which I assumed would soon reveal my condition, and, other than my doctors, two close friends, and, by chance, my massage therapist, the only person who knew, for months, was Tracey, whom I had sworn to secrecy.

I felt like a fraud.

I have made a career of teaching my students to prize the strength of vulnerability and the freedom of living with authenticity. *It takes courage and risk*, I often said, *but it's the path to true freedom and peace.* I believed this and I still do, but early in my Parkinson's journey, I could not practice what I preached.

---

1. Emerson, "Self-Reliance," 31.

A BETTER LIFE

Then, several things led me to disclose my disease publicly about eleven months after the diagnosis.

One was my inability, in my silence, to do anything positive with Parkinson's, which I desired and believed would be a key to finding meaning in having it. In order to do some good I had to be public. Another impetus for disclosure was the growing burden of my inauthenticity, the most difficult part being the message my silence would someday send to my students and, especially, to my children, whom I'd taught that honesty, integrity, and truth—particularly when facing adversity—are hallmarks of a life well lived.

Let me stress here that there are good reasons not to be public with an illness, and I do not judge anyone who keeps his or her condition private. In my case, however, the secrecy was destroying me.

Since becoming public, I have discovered that there are others like me, *many* others, in fact; and I am learning valuable lessons from living with this disease.

One key lesson is that people need each other in order to thrive, especially when we struggle. We are, in truth, fiercely *interdependent*, and living authentically, though it comes with risk, is crucial *because* it is so fundamentally human. As Camus somewhere put it, "But above all, in order to be, never try to seem." An authentic response to illness, which includes being vulnerable with and leaning on trusted others, is a path to healing, peace, and even newfound joy.

I am now a fifty-one-year-old with Parkinson's and life is still good. Different. Less certain. Accompanied by new challenges. But still good. What has it been like for me? How is it going? Thus far, mercifully slowly, the way all of the doctors assured me it would. In the three years since that fateful meeting with Dr. T, my physical challenges have become more noticeable and bothersome, at least to me, but they are not yet limiting. I have a tremor in my left index finger and left foot, which spreads to my arm and hand when I am cold or my adrenaline is up; and I have increasing stiffness in my left arm and hand. Also, my left arm doesn't hang or swing naturally when I stand, walk, or run; my left leg slightly drags sometimes, especially when I'm tired; and my ability to move fluidly ebbs and flows.

It seems safe to say that I will not realize my dream to pitch for the Houston Astros.

I have also lost a lot of my sense of smell; and I miss that—a lot. Some days I feel more fatigued than I used to, which my doctors point out might have as much to do with being in my fifties as it does with Parkinson's, and I get painful muscle cramps in my toes, feet, and legs—a condition called dystonia and a common Parkinson's symptom.

As my friend Michael Westphal puts it, Parkinson's makes you uncomfortable in your own body.

Still, I can do what I have always done. I swim and play basketball with my daughters, taxi them to school and to their acting, dance, piano, and art classes, and help with homework. I meet the demands of being a university administrator and professor, walk to meetings across the UT campus, teach my courses, and at home I do housework and yardwork. I run long distances and work out hard at the gym. I devote time and energy to the Michael J. Fox Foundation for Parkinson's Research and serve on the Board at Power for Parkinson's, an organization in central Texas, raising awareness and funding for Parkinson's research and care. I share an active, fully partnered life with my wife.

Limitations will come. This is how Parkinson's works.

On the whole, I have been able to calm my fears of a rapid physical decline because of my doctors' reassurances and the information available about the disease. What I have found to be a far greater challenge is dealing with the sadness, fear, and worry that come with an uncertain future. I was someone who had always been in control of my own body, had always been able to understand it, more or less. Parkinson's has altered that, too, and it is difficult to convey the enormity of this change.

LESSONS

Recently, I had the opportunity to run the New York City Marathon, my second marathon since learning I have Parkinson's three years ago. I'm still discerning what this extraordinary experience means to me, and what it is teaching me; when my family, many friends who are like family, my fellow Parkinson's journeyers, the Team Fox community, and a sea of anonymous faces and voices buoyed me with their chorus of support. Though I think of myself as one who can, if given enough time, find adequate words to express my thoughts and feelings, I admit that I am still working to find the words in this case.

But as I ran through a remarkable city on a picture-perfect day, with inexpressible joy prompted by seeing so many I love along the route, I reflected, as I tend to do, on some things I am learning and want to share.

Whether you struggle with Parkinson's disease, another chronic illness, or any hardship, I hope you will consider some of these lessons.

The beginning of your journey is difficult but arguably the most crucial part.

The thoughts and feelings you are having are normal and you will learn to tame them, especially as you share them with trusted others.

Your hardship can be an opportunity for growth, wisdom, and newfound meaning and joy.

We live as if we know a lot about the future when we do not, and all we have is today.

Living honestly and authentically with your struggles each day will make you stronger and more resilient, offer you peace, and can inspire other people.

There is great strength in vulnerability, and all of us are vulnerable.

You need others to support you, and they need you, too.

A serious illness certainly presents sizable challenges and losses. It can also lead to unexpected gains. For me, these gains have included deeper and more authentic relationships, reconciliation, personal growth, wisdom, deep gratitude, and newfound purpose, hope, and joy.

In this way, Parkinson's is my teacher. Its lessons unfold each day, little by little, through living life, enduring its setbacks, recognizing its beauty, and living out loud with Parkinson's and nurturing myself and others through more vulnerable and authentic love.

As the ancient Greek philosopher Epicurus suggests, "Do not spoil what you have by desiring what you have not; remember that what you now have was once among the things you only hoped for."[2]

---

2. Messer, ed., *The Sayings of Epicurus*, 1.

22

CHOOSING THE RIGHT DOCTOR

WHO IS YOUR DOCTOR?

When meeting another person with Parkinson's (PwP), it usually does not take long before someone asks, "So, who is your doctor?"

I suspect that this familiar practice stems from there being a shortage of neurologists trained as movement disorder specialists.[1] Because the pool in many locales is small, many of us are bound to share the same doctor. More significant, these inquiries seem also to follow from recognizing our common plight, our shared questions and struggles, while simultaneously affirming our solidarity. We stand with each other, those of us whom Parkinson's has tapped so rudely to join its club, interested in one another's well-being, eager to offer support, and stronger by virtue of our shared experience.

As is true with many chronic illnesses, when receiving a Parkinson's diagnosis and looking at the road ahead we do well to take the long view. In fact, we should plan for the need to manage our disease for many years, even decades, identifying and enlisting resources that will help sustain our physical, emotional, and relational health. To this end, nothing is more crucial or prudent than finding the right physicians. At their best, they stand in solidarity with us, helping us live as well as we can with what my diagnosing neurologist called "a new family member" that never leaves our presence.

---

1. See "Parkinson's disease: New drugs and treatments."

Although PwP require the care provided by a neurologist who, ideally, is a trained movement disorder specialist (MDS), we also need a general practitioner who attends to our broader health care needs. Some of us might need other specialists, too, and especially as the disease progresses. In all of our providers, we should look for and expect to have a relationship marked by at least these three essential qualities: *collaboration, communication*, and *compassion*.

COLLABORATION

Every physician-patient relationship should exhibit collaboration. Literally, to collaborate means to "co-labor" or to work together. This effort entails forming a partnership, with each person relying on one's expertise, experience, and wisdom to make vital contributions toward meeting shared goals. The physician has expertise in medicine and clinical practice, whereas the patient has expertise in living with Parkinson's and all the challenges this entails. The shared goal, of course, is helping the patient feel as well as possible for as long as possible.

The best physicians recognize these qualities of collaboration, value them, and uphold a commitment to them in every patient relationship. The best patients hold their physicians and themselves accountable for establishing and maintaining this unique partnership.

COMMUNICATION

For collaborative care to happen, physicians and patients need to communicate openly, equitably, and effectively. Openness requires honesty and candor; we should share everything that pertains to our health care needs. Equity plays out as physicians listen to patients at least as much as they speak to them. In fact, each expert collaborator needs to listen to the other's perspective in any office visit. The patient shares successes, challenges, and needs; the physician shares medical knowledge and clinical experience as part of a treatment plan. New insights present themselves as conversations and physical exams unfold. If a physician minimizes or otherwise dismisses the importance of listening closely to the expert partner, communication breaks down, collaboration ends, and care suffers.

COMPASSION

Perhaps more important than any other quality, compassion needs to pervade the physician-patient relationship. Offering another human being compassion, a term that literally means *suffer with*, must remain as the foundation of medical practice.

Although current medical education emphasizes physicians developing sound capacities for compassion (and for its close kin, empathy, which means, *to feel with*), historically physicians have too often been encouraged to practice with a degree of emotional separation or critical psychological distance in order to remain objective and scientific in their approach. The idea has been that emotional connections risk clouding clinical judgment.

However, good science and keen clinical skills go hand in hand with things like compassion and empathy, which are the opposite of separation and distance. Let us not forget that the Hippocratic Oath, which physicians affirm, states, "I will remember that there is art to medicine as well as science, and that warmth, sympathy, and understanding may outweigh the surgeon's knife or the chemist's drug."[2]

As philosopher and writer Albert Camus observed, "I have no idea what's awaiting me, or what will happen when this all ends. For the moment I know this: there are sick people and they need curing."[3] Those who live with illness surely need curing. We also need physicians who embrace collaboration, communication, and compassion.

If your relationship with your neurologist, your general practitioner, or other provider lacks any of these essential qualities, it might be time to take the longer view and consider a new doctor.

2. Shiel, "Medical Definition of Hippocratic Oath."

3. Camus, *The Plague*, 127.

23

SOJOURNING WITH LOSS

CHANGES

My friend Joe and I sit across from each other at a small table in a local coffee shop. We meet there every so often to catch up amid the quick pace of active lives. After a few minutes of talking about baseball, work, and family, Joe leans in and asks, "So, what's most difficult about having Parkinson's? I mean, what's the biggest change for you?"

To say that Joe is direct is like saying Texans enjoy barbecue.

As I enjoy what is left of my now faint ability to smell and take in the aromas wafting through the air, an internal voice considers responses to Joe's question.

Stiffness, slowness, labored dexterity, poor sleep, fatigue, knowing I have to take medicine four or more times a day for the rest of my life, managing these medicines' side effects, wondering if I can work until retirement age, worrying about the uncertainty of my new life—all of these changes come to mind. They have since that late October day when I learned my diagnosis.

INSIGHTS

Then, it hits me.

I look up and clear my throat.

"The most difficult part . . . is living with intense feelings of loss," I say.

Joe nods and takes a sip of his coffee.

I say, "Your body doesn't function like it used to. You do not feel as well as you once did. A sense of your overall well-being wanes. You have to let go of certain plans you have made for the future; or at least you have to reformulate them. You worry about burdening those you love most. You feel like you are living on borrowed time . . . and you know most of this will only get worse."

Again, he nods.

"It's like mourning a loved one's death . . . but it's the death of your former self. Parkinson's makes you have to figure out how best to live with that," I say.

Steam blows forcibly from an espresso machine before tapering to a gurgle.

"How do you do *that*?" Joe asks.

I have spent my professional life pondering this question, the question of how best to mourn.

As a doctoral student, I wrote a dissertation on elegiac poetry as a resource for complicated mourning. The poets, as Heidegger recognized, "reach into the abyss" to say what is true. For nearly two decades since, I have taught courses on loss and bereavement for budding therapists, ministers, and social workers. I have written articles on the subject and a couple of books as well, recognizing that, whether tied to illness or to a multitude of other factors—spouses, children, friendships, careers, dreams, or something else—losses eventually come to us *all* and we must find ways to live in their presence.

I am acutely aware of this universal human experience now. I live with it daily; so do most people who have a chronic illness. As Anne Lamott describes this living, "It's like having a broken leg that never heals perfectly—that still hurts when the weather gets cold, but you learn to dance with the limp."[1]

SOJOURNING

Returning to Joe's question, this is what I have learned about living with loss.

---

1. Lamott, *Plan B*, 174.

We mourn the loss of someone or something precisely because we have loved it; found meaning in it; derived pleasure from it; felt secure with it; and allowed it to become an integral part of us—a part of our identity.

As a result, we need never seek to forget, minimize, discount, or sever emotional ties with our losses. To do so is to deny, if not dishonor, both what we have lost and a part of ourselves. Instead, we can maintain these ties and nurture them in new ways. We do this by finding a new emotional space for what we lose. Speaking metaphorically, this space may hold our memories, gratitude, learnings, what we impart to others, our motivation to live more intentionally, or something else that keeps us firmly in relationship to our loss.

We can move our losses into this space, hold them there, and live consciously in their presence. We can sojourn with them; that is, stay with them temporarily, when we want or need to. Doing so allows for remembering our losses, but also forming and nurturing different, but still life-giving, relationships with what or whom we have loved.

Life endures amid our losses and illness. This I am learning, too. In the face of physical challenges, future uncertainty, questionable well-being—in the face of persistent losses—life still beckons us unceasingly to invest fully, love deeply, mourn actively, and never to opt for less.

As sojourners we learn, limp and all, how to dance again.

24

GETTING TO GRATEFUL

WHAT ARE YOU THANKFUL FOR?

It's bedtime for our young daughters. They have taken their baths, put on pajamas, and brushed teeth. Their mom and I have read a nightly lineup of books to them—*Goodnight Moon, Good Night Gorilla*, and, of course, *Good Night Texas*. The smell of lavender baby shampoo, lingering on still damp brown bangs that fall just above sleepy eyes, prompts my delight.

All of us now sit on Meredith's bed preparing for the last nightly ritual, something we began shortly after Holly was born and Meredith was two years old.

"Crisscross applesauce," Meredith says; a cue for us to sit up and cross our legs in a lotus-like position, which we do.

"I go first," Holly says, her pronounced dimples flanking a delicious smile.

"I go next," says Meredith, with bright, captivating eyes.

"Ready, Mommy?" Holly asks as Tracey smiles. ". . . What are you thankful for?"

We then each take turns speaking about our gratitude for what we have and experience.

"What are you thankful for?" has become our family bedtime refrain.

CHALLENGES TO GRATITUDE

I think a lot about gratitude these days. Three years ago, assuming I had lost nearly everything, I felt that my life more or less had ended with a Parkinson's diagnosis. I know that in similar circumstances many people feel this way.

There *have* been dark moments. After all, Parkinson's takes relentlessly from those it latches onto. Slowly, but surely. Over time, it can rob you of basic abilities: to move, to feel pleasure or calm, to sleep, and to speak, along with other aspects of life that I previously took for granted.

Perhaps you have taken them for granted, too. As Joni Mitchell observed, "Don't it always seem to go, that you don't know what you've got till it's gone."[1]

Gratitude can be elusive. When I labor to button my shirt with stiff fingers, it is difficult to feel thankful. On night four of waking up at 2 AM, unlikely to fall back asleep and anticipating a packed afternoon schedule, being grateful proves elusive. When, after a long day, I have painful cramping in my toes and feet—a condition called dystonia and a common Parkinson's symptom—gratitude remains a distant thought at best; just as it is when my legs feel like they have cinder blocks tied to them as I walk. It is difficult to maintain a posture of gratitude when life gets hard.

But what's a better alternative? Apathy? Bitterness? Despair?

No.

As Cicero observed, "Gratitude is not only the greatest of virtues, but the parent of all others."[2] As a result, we benefit from practicing gratitude as often as possible, and especially when facing challenges.

GETTING TO GRATEFUL

Here is what helps get me to a place of gratitude. This is how I practice it.

Name It

First, I *acknowledge* my hardships, which often involve the things I have lost or will never have. It is essential to recognize and affirm what causes pain, disappointment, anger, sadness, regret, fear, or any other feeling that

---

1. Morum and Mitchell, *Joni Mitchell*, 255.
2. Cicero, "Pro Plancio."

accompanies my struggles. In order to feel grateful, I must first recognize challenges to gratitude. Then, I must acknowledge them and the pain they cause. Otherwise, I will not heal. In order to answer the question, "What are you thankful for?" I first have to answer the question, "What is causing me pain?"

Claim It

Second, I have to *accept* what is happening. Having acknowledged my pain, I must next recognize that life will now be different. I'm not saying that I give up or that I live with resignation, only that I have to accept my situation as something that just has to be, perhaps forever, and that going forward life will not be the same as it was before. As Michael J. Fox points out, "Acceptance doesn't mean resignation; it means understanding that something is what it is and that there's got to be a way through it."[3]

Own It—All

Third, in order to feel grateful I focus on what I *do* have, on what I have *not* lost; including aspects of my life not diminished by having Parkinson's. Not only this, but, believe it or not, I focus further on the ways my life is *better* by virtue of living with this disease.

To be clear, I am not grateful I have Parkinson's. In fact, having it sucks. Big time. But having it has brought its own gifts that enrich my life beyond what I could have imagined.

I consider how my relationships have deepened and become more authentic; how my values have shifted; how my priorities have changed; how my hopes and dreams have morphed into more beautiful and life-giving possibilities; how I am graced by new friendships with those in the Parkinson's community.

Stephen Hawking, who lived an extraordinary life amid the cruel assault of ALS, puts it in perspective: "My expectations were reduced to zero when I was 21. Everything since then has been a bonus."[4]

3. Fox, "Michael J. Fox at 50."
4. Hawking, "The Science of Second-Guessing."

Gauge It

Finally, and this is tricky, my practice of gratitude includes a recognition of those whose hardships are much more severe than my own. I want to be careful here. Never would I hope to benefit from someone else's adversity or despair. In fact, I want to be a source of their comfort and joy.

At the same time, when I pay closer attention to others and truly empathize with their struggles, I often find that my own difficulties, though significant and worthy of the kind of acknowledgment I've suggested, nevertheless carry a magnitude of pain and suffering and despair that pales in comparison. Our mutual struggles bring us into solidarity, yes, *and* I remember the value found in the knowledge that "it can always be worse" and for some it already is.

PRACTICING THE REFRAIN

When the darker moments come, or when gratitude eludes me, I ask myself, "What are you thankful for?" Then, I look at what I have, or could have; at what enhances my life, relationships, sense of purpose and meaning, ability to support others, and new goals. I consider the abundance with which I live. Over and over, I practice this refrain.

Oliver Sacks was a renowned neurologist who pioneered the use of a drug called levodopa, a discovery that remains the gold standard for treatment of Parkinson's. He wrote a moving piece for the *New York Times* upon learning he had terminal cancer, in which he said, "I cannot pretend I am without fear. But my predominant feeling is one of gratitude. I have loved and been loved; I have been given much and I have given something in return; I have read and traveled and thought and written . . . Above all, I have been a sentient being, a thinking animal, on this beautiful planet, and that in itself has been an enormous privilege and adventure."[5]

I think of these words often, grateful that my own privilege and adventure continues.

5. Sacks, "My Own Life."

25

HOW DID YOU KNOW?

"HOW DID YOU KNOW?"

People ask me how I found out I have Parkinson's disease. This question never bothers me; no questions do, really. It is an unusual diagnosis to get in your late forties, and people are curious. I would be curious, too. I might even want reassurance that I did not have Parkinson's myself.

Getting my diagnosis required several things. One was paying attention to a faint tremor in my left index finger, but also listening to my gut. I knew something was not right with my body. A diagnosis also meant trusting my primary care doctor and following her advice, in spite of my fervent hope that it was overkill. After all, I had always been the picture of good health. Getting a diagnosis also required showing up for an appointment I never wanted to have, could easily have delayed, and for which I had to wait anxiously for over a month.

Ultimately, finding out I have Parkinson's required adhering to my belief that knowing the truth is better than running from it.

This is how I found out.

THE ERRATIC INDEX FINGER

In the fall of 2016, I sit comfortably at the cherry-colored wooden desk in my campus office. It's in the Steve Hicks School of Social Work at the

University of Texas at Austin, and I can look out of my window and see the university's iconic Tower and its Darrell K. Royal Memorial Stadium, where my favorite team since childhood, the Texas Longhorns, play football on Saturdays. Having lived in Texas as a child, pulling for the Texas Longhorns was my first religion.

As squealing bus brakes announce the arrival of students for early morning classes, I take quick sips of warm coffee between spurts of typing on my computer. With thoughts flowing, my excitement grows as something new begins to live on the page. My left hand, like my left wrist and forearm, has been stiff for months. It tries to keep pace with the right hand's fluid keystrokes.

A sudden twitch in my left index finger disrupts my work. Each time I extend it, like when reaching for the T key, it shakes quickly back and forth. You know how a parent shakes a finger when telling her child *No*, or not to do something? This is the kind of movement my finger is making. And I can't stop it. It does not move when at rest on the keyboard or desktop. But anytime I use it purposefully, like when typing or pointing at something, it swings back and forth like an erratic pendulum on a wall clock.

I chalk it up to having drunk too much coffee and don't think much more about it. But that afternoon it keeps twitching, and the same thing happens the next morning, and for the next few weeks.

Finally, I tell my wife about it. She encourages me to make an appointment with our doctor. I make the appointment and start Googling finger tremors.

I see my doctor and she refers me to a neurologist, Dr. T.

THE EXAM

On October 26, 2016, I meet Dr. T as he enters the exam room. A distinguished looking man in what I assume is his sixties, he has stylish wire-rimmed glasses and wears a purple bow tie, blue oxford shirt, and khaki pants. A burnt orange University of Texas lanyard hangs around his neck and holds his St. David's Medical Center ID badge.

He introduces himself, glances at the notes his nurse had taken a few minutes earlier, and then sits down at the small desk to my right.

"So, what's going on?" he says.

I tell him about the stiffness in my left forearm, wrist, hand, and fingers, making a fist several times as I speak.

"I have a tightness that won't go away and less dexterity in my fingers," I say.

He asks when I first noticed the change. I tell him it has been this way for at least six months, and probably longer, and that I especially notice it when writing and typing.

"I'm left handed," I say.

Then, I show him the tremor in my left index finger. As he moves closer to look for the faint twitch, I quickly emphasize how active I am, how I tend to push myself at the gym.

"I have probably been overdoing it in my workouts. I've been known to do that," I say.

His eyes inspect my body as I speak. He looks like a detective at a crime scene. I worry that the crime scene is my body.

"I saw Dr. W a few weeks ago. She thought it would be a good idea for me to see you," I tell him.

With pursed lips, he nods in agreement, still looking me over with his Columbo eyes.

Despite thinking there's a chance I have Parkinson's, given the previous diagnosis of physiologic tremor I'm betting he'll perform a brief examination, tell me to dial it back at the gym, maybe order physical therapy, and then wish me well as he sends me on my way. After all, I have always been healthy and I take good care of myself.

He reaches into his weathered black leather doctor's bag and says, "Let's take a look," as he directs me to an exam table. I climb up on it and he begins his work.

Holding up his index finger, he asks me to follow it with my eyes. As he moves it to different places, I track: left, right, up, down, straight ahead, then back to the left, up, down. He then asks me to reach out and touch the tip of his finger with each of my index fingers, first the left one, then the right one, again moving his finger to different places every time there's contact. He also has me touch the tip of my nose with both of my index fingers, sort of like a field sobriety test for suspected drunk drivers.

Next, he checks my reflexes in several places, has me tap my fingers together and tap my feet to the floor in different combinations, and then asks me to push and pull with my hands against his resistance. With earnestness, I follow his commands. After this, he takes a metal instrument from his bag. Sliding it down my shins, he asks if I could feel the sensation. I can. It feels cold.

When he finishes with my shins, he points to the small desk beside the exam table.

"Have a seat over there," he says.

When I sit down, he gives me a pen and a piece of paper and asks me to write something, which I do. My left wrist and forearm move with deliberateness as I write. As has been the case for several months, my hand-writing is labored and messy.

When I finish, he gestures with his arm and asks me to follow him.

We leave the exam room and step into a long hallway with bare beige walls; their nakedness aligns with a growing emptiness in my chest. He asks me first to walk toe to heel in a straight line, and then to walk naturally down to the end of the hallway and back. As I will later learn, he is checking my balance, arm swing, and gait—all part of the standard exam protocol for Parkinson's disease and other movement disorders.

When I finish, we return to the exam room and he asks me to sit on the table again. Giving sustained attention to my left side, he rechecks the reflexes in my elbow and ankle, and also rotates each back and forth.

"How am I doing?" I ask.

He offers no response but keeps looking at my left elbow. He taps it a few more times with the dark orange rubber head of a reflex hammer.

THE LIFE-CHANGING WORDS

For a moment, I wonder if he is this thorough with all of his patients, but then the pensive look on his face signals that something is wrong. He gives my elbow one more tap. Then, with a slightly furrowed brow, he invites me to return to the chair beside the desk.

He sits down, too, and leans toward me.

"What worries me is that I think you are in the early stages of Parkin-son's disease," he says.

I feel my throat closing and it's hard to breathe. I feel hot all over my body and it's tough to sit still.

He opens up a black three-ring binder that he has pulled from the desk drawer. With pages of diagnostic information about Parkinson's, he turns it my way as he begins to explain its contents.

He tells me that Parkinson's follows from a loss of neurons in the brain that produce dopamine, a neurotransmitter that affects the body's ability for movement and experiencing reward. He then shows me a diagram of where this all goes down, pointing to an area in the brain called the *basal ganglia* and, more specifically, the *substantia nigra*. His notebook holds drawings, tables, charts, and lists. Each protected by a plastic sheet. Each blurred as I attempt to follow along.

"These are the criteria we look at when you present with Parkinson's symptoms," he says, pointing to one of the lists.

I see in bold type: *Bradykinesia (slowness of movement) must be present with one or more of the following: muscular rigidity, tremor, or postural instability.*

"If someone has at least two of these symptoms, and you do—bradykinesia and rigidity—we make the diagnosis," he says.

When I finally speak, my voice cracks like a pubescent teenager.

"But I have young children . . . How will I tell my parents . . . ? How sure are you about this?"

"I'm pretty sure," he says.

"But how do you know?" I ask.

THE EVIDENCE

"Several things are going on. You have slowness on your left side, and this is what we look for first. You also have rigidity in your wrist and arm. The arm does not have a natural swing to it when you walk; and when I move your wrist back and forth, it is not a fluid motion but, instead, has what we call cogwheeling. It almost clicks when you move it, like a ratchet wrench," he says.

I stare at him blankly as my mind flashes back a few weeks, to when my kids and I rode boogie boards for hours in Surfside Beach, South Carolina, and when all seemed right in the world and there were smiles and freedom to savor.

Silence.

"We've only just met, and you might be a serious guy, but your face shows what we call masking; it takes on a more serious look than it had before and shows less expression. It's a common early symptom . . . and while it's very subtle in your case, I know what to look for, and I can see it."

He closes his notebook and breaks another block of silence by saying he wants me to have an imaging test.

"I want you to have something called a DaTscan. I rarely order this because the diagnosis can typically be made from the exam. But you're young to have Parkinson's and your symptoms are subtle. The scan will let us know for sure," he says.

I keep staring at him, wondering if I will walk my children down the aisle at their weddings, or if I'll even be at their weddings. I reach down and grab the seat of my hard wooden chair with sweaty hands.

"This will progress slowly. It is likely going to be at least ten, maybe fifteen years before you notice significant changes, and maybe even longer. I'll see you a couple of times a year; and I suspect that every year or so you'll report the symptoms are getting a little worse and the exam will show that, too. That's how it typically goes for younger people."

He pauses to let me catch up. I wonder how many of these conversations he's had over the years.

"I've been doing this for a long time. We know how to treat this disease, and we *are* on the verge of real breakthroughs. Many new treatments are on the horizon . . . I would not have said this a few years ago, but I honestly believe that we'll soon have good options for new kinds of treatment—better treatments; and there's real hope that we are close to finding a way to stop, and maybe even reverse, the progression."

I try to absorb his words. Try to hope.

"I want you to remember something. It's really important. People experience the disease differently. It's not the same for everyone," he says.

He pauses, looks me in the eye with a Texan's directness and authenticity, and then says, "This disease is different for everyone. Don't let someone else's story become your story."

At the time, I did not understand the importance of this advice.

THE NEW KIND OF LIFE

The appointment concludes with him handing me a prescription for Azilect, an MAO-B inhibitor, and some samples, which he tells me to start taking immediately. I had learned that this drug prevents an enzyme in your brain from breaking down the dopamine you still have, so that you hold on to it for longer. He asks me to return in one month and encourages me to bring Tracey.

He says, "I know this is hard, Allan. There's a lot to take in. You now have a new family member. Everywhere you go, you will take that family member with you. It will take some time to adjust."

I can only imagine the look on my face, but Dr. T must sense that I am still processing his revelations. He pauses again. Then, he reiterates what he has just said.

"I would like you to come back next month with your wife. You'll both have questions and I want to do my best to answer them."

Still sitting in the exam room chair, I look down at the faint tremor in my left index finger, the reason for my initial appointment with my primary care doctor and a symbol for a new kind of life. Dr. T opens the door and waits for me to stand. I see those naked hallway walls, which now align with my heart.

He extends his hand and shakes mine. We walk together to the front desk area, where patients pay their bills and make their next appointments. My stomach churns, and my legs feel like they might not hold me up. When we arrive there, his eyes again lock with mine. He places his hand on my shoulder and repeats his advice.

Remember, don't let someone else's story become your story.

I nod my head, still trying to take it all in. I manage to get out a soft *thank you* as he turns and walks away.

After scheduling my follow-up appointment, I leave the office, walking slowly toward the parking garage as the world whirls by. Somehow, I find my way back to my car as questions, thoughts, and feelings ricochet through my malfunctioning brain and body.

I open my car's door, sit down, and weep.

As I drive home, I keep thinking, *But I have young children . . .*

26

FACES OF HUMANITY

LOSING FACE

"We've only just met, and you might be a serious guy, but your face shows what we call masking; it takes on a more serious look than it had before and shows less expression," he says.

I nod as my blank stare meets his earnest eyes. Reaching down, I grab the seat of my chair to steady myself as the exam room whirls and spins.

Then he says, "It's a common early symptom . . . and while it's very subtle in your case, I know what to look for, and I can see it."

Dr. T, a neurologist to whom my primary care doctor has referred me, speaks these words as he diagnoses me with Parkinson's disease at the age of forty-eight.

I can only imagine the look on my face.

A few months later, I walk from my campus office to a nearby classroom where a small production team awaits. We are filming a new video for the Steve Hicks School of Social Work at The University of Texas at Austin, where I work as a professor and academic dean. As the production team finishes filming me, the producer says, "I really like what you said, but could you do it again with more expression in your face?" I keep trying to do what he asks, and hark back to my meeting with Dr. T. After three takes, with my increasing efforts to be animated, the producer says, "Much better! I think we've got what we need."

Still locked in the Parkinson's closet, my body will slowly reveal my secret and I can do nothing to stop it.

Those who have Parkinson's tend to lose some of their ability for facial expression, which has numerous implications. We can take on a more serious appearance, such that people wonder if we are sad or angry. Over time, we may blink less often and may seem to stare coldly at people or things we love; and sometimes people mistakenly assume that a flatter face correlates with a depressive state, diminished cognition, or less facility with carrying on a conversation.

The mask Parkinson's forces us to wear is a cruel one. When we feel intensely and desperately want to share our emotions, we might be incapable.

THE SIGNIFICANCE OF FACES

The first time I recall thinking in any sustained way about the human face was in graduate school, in a course on the theories of developmental psychologist Erik H. Erikson. He wrote about the earliest interactions between an infant and primary caregivers, and of the powerful effect that their faces have on the baby. A kind, responsive, and empathic face conveys love, nurture, and hope. Over time, and when joined to consistent offers of support for meeting the infant's needs, these face-to-face encounters help the infant develop a sense of being valued, safe, and deserving of benevolent care, qualities that then become the infant's own and shape his or her sense of self.

This dynamic of interpersonal exchange continues as we age and mature. We cultivate and develop these same vital qualities in face-to-face encounters with trusted others at any age and throughout life.

In my forties, I read the work of the French philosopher Emmanuel Levinas, who offered his own take on the importance of faces. He said that another person's face, when we encounter it, makes an ethical claim on us that bids us to take responsibility for how we treat one another. For Levinas, "the face is the most exposed, most vulnerable, and most expressive aspect of the other's presence . . . [The] face speaks to me and thereby invites me to a relation."[1] Moreover, another's face "offers itself to [my] compassion and [my] obligation."[2] As noted previously, face-to-face encounters, it turns

---

1. Levinas, *Totality and Infinity*, 198.
2. Robins, ed., *Is It Righteous to Be?*, 48.

out, change us; they humanize us because they obligate us to one another, calling us to become the best version of human we can become.

Looking in the mirror, I can see that, in a sense, I am losing face with Parkinson's. The changes are subtle, as Dr. T said, but they will likely intensify with time. I wonder what Levinas would say about this loss.

I know that despite losses to the "most expressive aspect of my presence," I feel more human than I ever have—more vulnerable and exposed, yes, less attractive and desirable, perhaps, but also more authentic and real, open and connected, daring and alive. Whatever role vanity played in my life previously, Parkinson's has challenged and diminished it. Michael J. Fox was right when he said that with Parkinson's you have to throw vanity out the window. Doing so has been much easier than I would ever have imagined. Although I'm still self-conscious about the effects of Parkinson's on my physical appearance, maybe Janis Joplin was right, too, when she said that freedom is just another word for nothing left to lose.[3]

LIVING FACE TO FACE

On the one hand, we put too much emphasis on faces, and especially on improving and maintaining them, which requires a lot of emotional energy. We fret over them becoming wrinkled, blemished, or less supple than they once were. We spend lots of money on trying to make them more attractive, with products and even surgeries, striving to reach norms of beauty that our society tells us are ideal but, in fact, are unreachable. Women often bear the heaviest burdens related to these norms and social expectations, but men suffer from the weight as well.

At the same time, faces often are not ascribed the status they deserve. Genetically, human beings are 99.9 percent similar, but science has confirmed the singular status of every human face. In fact, a prevailing theory holds that, over time, human faces evolved with differences for a particular reason, namely so that we may tell each other apart. Different faces reflect our standing as unique persons.

Too frequently, we do not see faces for what they are, namely, a one-of-a-kind reflection of something mysterious, valuable, and sacred; a numinous expression of one who encounters us and changes us. At least I have not always seen faces this way. As a result, my face-to-face encounters have

3. Joplin, "Me and Bobby McGee."

been less frequent, less valued, and more rushed than I want them to be. Too often, a phone call, email, or text message has replaced them.

My doorbell rings. It's a warm Sunday afternoon in the fall of 2017. I peer out our front bay window and there stands my friend Robert. A tall man, he has a warm smile and piercing blue eyes. We have known each other for several years, ever since our kids were in preschool, but it's been months since we've seen each other. He is also a professor at UT, and we both live with crammed schedules.

I open the front door and see that he has ridden his bike, which he has leaned against our front gate. A devoted father, the trailer bike attached to his bike often holds one of his children. But today he's by himself.

He says, "I've been thinking about you and I decided to ride over and say hello." Unannounced and uninvited, his visit reminds me of the way it is with kids, and of how it used to be among grown-ups, and it makes my day. I tell my Tracey about this visit and pledge to follow Robert's example of dropping by unannounced for a visit with friends, for no other reason than that they are on my mind.

Four months later, I would attend his memorial service after he suffered a massive stroke and died.

I no longer take any face for granted. Actually, I want to see more faces, more often and more authentically.

I want others to see my face, too, even if what they see is less expressive than I would like.

Seizing opportunities for more empathy, love, and hope, more compassion and obligation—just as Erikson and Levinas said can happen when we come face to face with each other—I am becoming more human.

27

LENSES OF STRENGTH

DISABILITY

When does one assume the status of disabled? I have thought about this question since my Parkinson's diagnosis over three years ago. The Americans with Disabilities Act (ADA) says it is when a physical or mental impairment substantially limits one or more major life activities.[1] It turns out that over 61 million American adults, or one in four, live with at least one type of disability. Some live with multiple types. Six forms of disability, listed in order of prevalence, include movement, cognition, hearing, vision, independent living, and self-care.[2] Worldwide, 15 percent of the population, or 1 billion people, live with one or more of these disabilities.[3]

A vexing issue around disability is how often those of us with defined conditions that are associated with disability, such as Parkinson's, are kept out of the game even if our tryouts are excellent. In fact, many people view disabled persons through a lens of deficits as opposed to strengths, and these people see what they assume those who are disabled *cannot* do as opposed to what they *can* do.

1. See "What is the definition of disability under the ADA?"
2. See "CDC 1 in 4 US Adults Live with a Disability."
3. See "World Report on Disability."

WHAT DISABLED PERSONS OFFER

Studies have shown that persons with disabilities can actually do a lot. For example, when businesses make hiring people with disabilities a priority, they outperform businesses that do not.[4] Disability-friendly businesses had 28 percent higher revenues, their net income was twice as much as other businesses, and their profit margins were 30 percent higher.[5] Moreover, the U.S. Department of Labor found that disability-friendly employers had a 90 percent increase in employee retention.[6]

Having disabled persons in the workplace also fosters a culture of empathy and support, which benefits everyone. Non-disabled persons become more aware of how to make the workplace more inclusive. Disabled persons contribute distinct insights, perspectives, and wisdom born of resilience, discipline, and typically a strong work ethic. Because persons with disabilities must constantly adapt to their surroundings, they also bring creativity, agility, persistence, openness, forethought, and capacity for solving problems.[7] Hiring disabled workers makes good sense.

FRUSTRATION

My friend Eric recently had an experience of colleagues seeing disability through the lens of deficits and he steamed with frustration. After interviewing the last of four candidates who had applied for a senior staff position in the university's library, he and his colleagues met to discuss the applicants and make a recommendation to their dean.

Eric said, "We were discussing the candidates and deliberating about whom to recommend for hire. Although none of the first three stood out, this last candidate was outstanding—bright, experienced, visionary. But he had a form of Asperger's, and my fellow committee members made some horrible remarks. They said he could not be trusted to represent the library, that he would speak without thinking, and some other critical things about his disability. The Deputy University Librarian just sat there and did not say anything. I spoke up and kept trying to persuade them, but the others dismissed me. It was painful and embarrassing."

4. "Getting to Equal."
5. "Getting to Equal."
6. "Getting to Equal."
7. "Getting to Equal."

BUILDING AN INCLUSIVE COMMUNITY

Despite the too-common approach of avoiding disabled persons, innovative advocates are creating new models. A couple of decades ago, I discovered Jean Vanier, a philosopher, theologian, and humanitarian who died earlier this year. For over half a century, he advocated for persons living with developmental and intellectual disabilities, going so far as to establish communities in which they may live full and dignified lives. Vanier's work began in the early 1960s, when, having moved from his native Canada to France, he visited a psychiatric hospital located in a southern suburb of Paris. He met two men who resided there, and their personal distress and poor living conditions disturbed him. As Vanier put it, they lived walled off from the world, their humanity unrecognized.

Seeking a way to change their situation and to offer them a more supportive and dignified life, his solution was to welcome these two men into his home and to become their caregiver, which he did in 1964. Soon thereafter, his care for persons with disabilities broadened when he founded a residential community in the same town. He called it L'Arche, which, in English, means the Ark.

Vanier and the L'Arche community offered disabled persons living in institutions a different kind of life, one in which they were treated as full human beings with dignity. Vanier recognized not only their humanity; he also saw their ability to teach us about being human. In particular, he saw that "the weak teach the strong to accept and integrate the weakness and brokenness of their own lives."[8] Embodying this insight, Vanier devoted his life to building communities of hospitality and support for disabled people and their families all around the world. His work continued until his death earlier this year (2019), at the age of ninety. Today, there are 153 L'Arche communities in thirty-eight countries on five continents.[9]

EDUCATING AND ADVOCATING

Which brings me to Sean Pevsner.

It is just after noon when he rolls into the classroom in a wheelchair he controls with his head. The soft hum of the electric motor breaks the

---

8. Vanier, *The Scandal of Service*, 2.

9. Vanier's biographical information may be found at http://www.jean-vanier.org.

otherwise lengthy silence. I cannot tell whether those in the audience are surprised, uncomfortable, or in awe.

Sean was born with severe cerebral palsy. Now in his mid-forties and a civil rights attorney, he is at The University of Texas at Austin's Steve Hicks School of Social Work to kick off a speaker series for Disability Awareness Month. He has difficulty speaking, so his personal aid helps him communicate using a combination of human interactions and technological tools.

Sean's presentation begins with a video telling his story through images of his life and work. Photos of him in the hospital as a child, going to elementary school, graduating from college and then from law school, and preparing and trying cases flash across the screen, as do shots of him lobbying the Texas legislature on behalf of persons with disabilities. As the video plays, a computer-generated narrator speaks Sean's words for him.

He recounts obstacles he has faced as well as how he got around them. One obstacle was when he and his parents fought for the right to attend mainstream classes in the Arlington (Texas) Public Schools, which resulted in him being among the first students with disabilities to do so. He also speaks at length about the hard work it took to convince the Texas Bar Association to let him take the bar exam after completing his studies at the UT School of Law. He recounts how, through the years, some attorney colleagues and even judges have dismissed his ability to represent his clients effectively; on several occasions, they even sought to have him removed from cases. The title of his address could not have fit more perfectly with the purpose of this event: "Be Your Own Advocate."

Afterwards, several people in the audience ask him questions. One person, a UT law professor, inquires about how he kept from getting discouraged, especially when practicing law and advocacy in a state that, historically, has not had the political will to fund or provide adequate services to those living with disabilities. This professor even singles out a couple of long-term politicians and their poor records on this front. Many in the audience nod in agreement.

Silence fills the room as Sean thinks for a moment. Then he begins communicating with his aide, who listens to Sean as he types on a device that looked like a large iPad. When they finish, and after checking the accuracy of what he has typed, the aide reads Sean's response as he smiles with bright eyes and a toothy grin.

"I never back down from a fight."

LENSES OF STRENGTH

The world needs more people like my friend Eric, Jean Vanier, and Sean Pevsner. Living into the fullness of our humanity depends on it. We might not choose to launch communities such as L'Arche or have to overcome the types of obstacles Sean faces, but we can challenge those who see disabled persons through lenses of deficit to begin seeing through lenses of strength. As Eric did, we can also speak out against discrimination, exclusion, and, perhaps, downright meanness. Like Sean, we can educate people, disabled and non-disabled alike, and bid them to consider new perspectives. As Jean did, we can affirm the dignity of every human being, including those who live with disabilities, and recognize that disabled persons can do many things well and even have unique contributions to make.

I find myself believing that, upon seeing a man with severe cerebral palsy practicing law, Vanier would say, "See! The weak teach the strong!" To which Pevsner might say, "Yes, but the weak are strong, too; and there may be times when we have to fight, for others and ourselves, for what is fair, equitable, and just."

28

TWO QUESTIONS

THE PHONE CALL

I am in the middle of getting a massage when the phone rings. My doctor had suggested this given the stiffness in my left forearm, wrist, and hand. Normally I would have the phone turned off, but nothing about my life on this day feels normal. I am anticipating this call from my neurologist, Dr. T, and I want to get it over with, to have confirmation of something I already know in my gut.

My massage therapist excuses herself from the room.

"Hello," I say.

"Hi, Allan. This is Dr. T. We got the results from the scan, and, unfortunately, it confirms what we discussed. You do have Parkinson's disease."

Silence.

"I see . . . Well . . .what do I do now?" I say.

"Like we discussed, take your medicine and come see me in a month," he says.

The call ends and I place my phone back on the small table, next to my glasses, wallet, and car keys. I climb back on the massage table in only my boxer shorts and get under the sheet. I welcome its warmth against my chilled soul. Meditative music plays softly behind my head. A small candle that I am certain smells good burns beside me. Parkinson's has already taken much of my ability to smell. Maybe it's vanilla-scented, which I love; and, I think to myself, *Before I leave, I will put my nose really close to that candle.* Lying on my back, I stare at the ceiling with my hands under my head. I have had fantasies about Dr. T's call going differently than it did, and yet I'm not surprised by the news.

I say it in my head in different ways: *I* have Parkinson's disease. I *have* Parkinson's disease. I have *fucking Parkinson's disease.*

I invite my massage therapist back into the room, but echoes of the phone call are still in my head.

What do I do now?

ACCESSING MYSELF

I have always been a doer, and a thinker. In fact, I have lived as though I can *do* or *think* my way toward achieving almost anything; and it has often worked. The challenge has been to allow myself to *feel.* Not to feel for *others*—I am pretty compassionate and empathic—but to feel for *myself*; to feel my *own* losses, disappointments, and fears; and especially to risk being vulnerable enough to share them. Access to these feelings has always been restricted, if not to myself, certainly to others. Tracey pointed this out to me more than twenty-five years earlier. Having Parkinson's would change this. It would increase my tolerance for finding and sharing my more difficult feelings.

Dostoevsky said, "The mystery of human existence lies not in just staying alive, but in finding something to live for."[1] For months after my diagnosis, merely staying alive consumed me. Naively assuming I would soon approach a kind of Parkinson's cliff, only to fall off it into the abyss, I spent many days and most nights obsessed with self-preservation. I read about the latest research, evaluated the most effective medication protocols, located the best centers of care, and explored various exercise programs, diets, and approaches to self-care. These efforts are valuable and I still spend time on them, but initially they rose from a place of intense fear and desperation. This meant I fixated on maintenance, and not growth; on the future, and not the present; on staying alive, and not on living.

In fact, I needed to rediscover what I would live for.

---

1. Dostoevsky, *The Brother's Karamazov,* 339.

WHAT AND HOW

Early one morning, I watch the sunrise as I run around Lady Bird Lake, near my home in Austin. Struggling with this fear and desperation, knowing that my life will include Parkinson's disease, I ask myself two questions. *What matters most to me?* and *How do I want to spend my time?*

I realize that what matters most are being a reliable and ethical person—as a husband, father, son, friend, colleague, neighbor, and citizen—and furthering compassion, justice, and love. I realize, too, that I want to spend my time doing something good with Parkinson's, such as educating, advocating, and writing about my own Parkinson's journey in order to build solidarity and form deeper connections with others.

I needed to name it as explicitly as I could. After all, it is what I am living for.

TELL ME

Life changes with a chronic illness, but a life with Parkinson's is still a life. It simmers with challenges, some of which are significant, but amid these challenges it also boils over with opportunities—new opportunities for meaningful, rewarding, compassionate, and generous experiences and relationships, within the Parkinson's community and beyond.

Whether you live with Parkinson's or not, if you have not yet done so I urge you to get going on your new life road. Reconnect, recommit, renew, and remind yourself of your passions, your dreams, and your purpose as best you can figure it out for now. Everyone is on the clock—every one of us. Keep this in mind.

29

WE HAVE OUR SHIT AND EACH OTHER

"Life might prove difficult—was evidently going to; but meanwhile they had each other, and that was everything."

—Henry James[1]

BEFORE I KNEW

I meet John at the gym one Monday morning at 6 AM, and both of us have a cup of coffee in our hand and sleepiness in our eyes. My wife and our daughters have given me personal training sessions as a Father's Day gift. I have worked out religiously for decades, since I was a teenager, in fact, but I am mostly self-taught and have never worked with a personal trainer.

When we shake hands, the veins in John's right biceps pop out like a small train tunnel, temporarily altering the multicolored pattern of tattoos that cover his entire arm. Pleasant but not enthusiastic, he appears mid-twentyish and has a wide smile that pushes out from his heavy beard.

We spend a few minutes going over the program he put together for me after our initial consultation the previous week. I then warm up by joining two dozen others on rows of elliptical machines, all of us pursuing

1. James, *The Wings of the Dove*, 69.

better fitness and most, I suppose, hoping to fend off the effects of advancing years. Ten minutes later, John returns and begins leading me through a series of exercises.

Most are familiar and I can complete them without too much effort; after all, I have always been athletic.

Then we get to the walking lunges.

When I lunge forward with my right leg, I feel shaky and off-balance. Though it's subtle, I sense it. I think I must need a longer warm-up, so I jog in place and stretch my legs—first, my hamstrings, then my quadriceps—and I keep reattempting the lunges, trying to compensate for the wobbliness each time I step out with my right leg.

As I lunge, sway, and jerk to recover and realign myself, I look like a young horse learning to walk. After a couple of additional wobbly attempts, I look back at John.

"See what you have to look forward to?" I say.

He smiles. "Keep going!"

"Approaching fifty isn't for the faint of heart!" I say.

He pushes out a one-syllable chuckle while nodding his head.

"You'll want to keep working on those lunges," he says.

"You *think?*"

This makes him laugh.

After a few more unsteady attempts, we move to another exercise, and then to several others, and I continue to meet with him until I finish my six sessions.

The wobbling continues.

John says nothing more about it.

I attribute it to my pushing fifty.

Months later, I would learn I have Parkinson's disease.

A few months after that, I would learn that John had died.

By suicide.

NOW THAT I KNOW

With the gift of hindsight, I wish I could go back to my last training session with John and say something like this.

I will soon learn that I have Parkinson's disease, John, and its burdens will be my life struggle.

My wife Tracey often reminds me that at any moment in time we can rightly assume that people we know and love, as well as those we have just met, face difficulties in their lives. Whether they share it or not, and even when smiles cover sadness, or humor hides fear, or work numbs pain, the struggles are there—real, hard, and sometimes life-threatening.

You'd have to know her to appreciate this fully, but Tracey says, "Everyone has their shit!"

Maybe it is a relationship, or finances, or a job, or Parkinson's, or depression, or some other hardship, but everyone has their shit!

Or they will.

Even so, what we also have, and we don't always know it, is a chance for connection. I wish I could have offered you more connection in the struggle, and that maybe you could have done that for me, too, once I knew what I would be dealing with. I know there is no guarantee that things would have been different. But I do know there is a chance that the more willing we are to share the dark places and our hardships, the more likely it is we can find some light.

John, we need one another.

We need to give and receive offers of kindness and compassion, in words and gestures. Sometimes we need to forgive or to be forgiven. We need to let go of harsh critiques and judgment, of others and of ourselves. We need to give each other the benefit of the doubt, see one another through appreciative eyes, and see ourselves in a similar way. We need to remind ourselves that we're all in this life together, as shit-filled as it gets.

We have each other.

The next time I am at the gym, I will do some walking lunges and think about John.

30

DEAR OZZY, KEEP DREAMING!

Dear Ozzy,

It's 1981, and I'm in the eighth grade. I spend a lot of time in my basement listening to your new record, *Diary of a Madman*. My friends and I love it; a couple of us have even been sounding out power chords on our guitars as we listen and play along. We have listened to *Blizzard of Oz*, your first record, for nearly a year, when playing basketball and talking about girls and Mustangs. Who doesn't love to jam to "Crazy Train"?

But what you might not know is that your music also speaks to our adolescent angst and gives us hope. Ours is an awkward phase of life. We are trying to moderate hormones and new kinds of urges, wanting to be kids and grown-ups simultaneously. We are trying to figure out who we are and who we want to be. You help us with all of that, and we dream of seeing you live when you come back to Atlanta.

Fast forward to 2020.

I am now almost fifty-two, and I learned yesterday that, like me, you have Parkinson's disease. I'm sorry, Ozzy, to have to welcome you to the "family." But I'm also glad you're here if it has to be this way. After all, as you will see, it is a stunningly generous and supportive family to join.

One thing you learn about Parkinson's is that it's different for everyone. Symptoms differ, as do the particular challenges that come with it. In fact, it is sort of like people who dig rock and roll. Some gravitate toward you, others toward AC/DC, still others toward Led Zeppelin, and some of us like all three and more. But as different as Parkinson's can be among those who have it, there's a lot we have in common. I could never have imagined the immediate bond you can feel with another human for no other reason than you share the same sinister disease. You will see this if you have not already.

At any rate, I don't want to be presumptuous, but I thought I'd reach out and offer a few things you might think on in these days; some gentle advice if you will. You helped me during my awkward years. Maybe I can help you now.

Take a slow, deep breath. It's going to be OK. Life will change, certain things will become more challenging, you will need to make managing your Parkinson's a priority, but this disease is treatable for most people; its symptoms can be managed for a long time. It tends to progress slowly. Your life expectancy is essentially what it would be if you did not have Parkinson's. Remind yourself of this and live your life accordingly.

Find your people. I mentioned the Parkinson's family. It is important to meet, spend time with, lean on, and learn from others who live with the Parkinson's beast. I cannot stress enough how much of a difference it makes to have your people who "get it" because they "have it." I know you must have many questions. I think we all do when embarking on this new life road. Having friends with Parkinson's whom I can reach out to, at any time, to ask questions, draw encouragement, and learn from has proven invaluable. You might need some folks to talk you off the ledge occasionally, too.

Keep moving. My neurologist said this to me as I left my first appointment with him, and it is sound advice. We know that regular vigorous exercise not only helps those with Parkinson's feel better, and move better, but it also helps slow down disease progression. It does not really matter what you do to keep moving, whether it's running, swimming, biking, boxing, yoga, tai chi, dancing, or something else. Just find something you like, or keep doing what you already do and enjoy, and it will serve you well over the long haul.

Slow down but speed up. Speaking of long hauls, remember to strike a balance between slowing down to enjoy what is most important to you, and speeding up so that you cease to delay experiences that you find meaningful. Parkinson's helps you not take as much for granted because it takes so much from you. You learn to value what you have, to see it more clearly, and to relish in the awareness that nothing lasts forever, for anyone. All of us are on the clock, Ozzy, whether we have Parkinson's or not. All we have is today, and we damn well should make the most of it. There is freedom in living with this awareness.

I am a teacher, and so I could go on and on, but here are a couple more suggestions.

Use your Parkinson's for good in the world. Having a chronic illness is hard, but you can find meaning in it and help others do the same if you use it as the basis for growth and enlightenment, generosity and compassion, kindness and even joy. I don't know what any of that will look like for you, and perhaps you do not yet know either, but you will figure it out if you keep it in mind and hold it to be a high value. You have a platform and voice that few people have, Ozzy. It is exciting to imagine how you will use these for good, and not just with respect to Parkinson's.

Keep dreaming big dreams. In your song "Dreamer" you say, "I'm just a dreamer, who dreams of better days." You have Parkinson's, but you also have a life to live, people to love, songs to write and record, and shows to perform. And it might be hard to believe this, but you will have better days ahead. You will have worse days, too. That's how it is with Parkinson's. But still, dare to dream, Ozzy. It keeps us all alive.

I saw you and Sharon interviewed by Robin Roberts on *Good Morning America*. It is clear how much you love one another. It is also clear that your marriage is marked by mutual devotion. This, too, is a gift and will provide you with a measure of power and hope that you will need. Indeed, I cannot imagine doing Parkinson's without my amazing wife, Tracey. I also could not help but notice how moved Sharon became when asked what she would want your fans to know. Talking about how much you love to perform, and how much you love your fans, she echoed your statement that your fans are the air that you breathe. You said, "I need them."

We are here for you, Ozzy, and those of us in the Parkinson's community need you, too. Together, we dream of better days.

Your fan,

Allan

P.S. Here's an idea. How about an Ozzfest for Parkinson's? We could have the first one here in Austin, Texas, which, as you know, is a great music town. And we have bats!

31

ON THE CLOCK

EARLY

It's early in the morning, and I'm at Baylor Scott and White Rehab going through the exercises that Sierra, my physical therapist (PT) has prescribed. She and I have been working together for several weeks as I try to strengthen my glutes, loosen my IT band, and fend off the episodic pain in my left knee. When you get a Parkinson's diagnosis, your doctors stress the importance of having a PT on your care team. Yes, for most of us, it takes a team of health care providers, or it will, to maintain our quality of life—to keep us moving, sleeping, speaking, and functioning in the ways that any human desires and most take for granted.

My focus is training for a marathon, which is still several weeks away. Exercise remains my Parkinson's drug of choice.

I engage in the movements that the PT exercise requires, with my glutes on fire and my core engaged, rep after rep, set after set. A woman about my age works with a different PT doing neck exercises, while an older man rehabs his freshly replaced knee.

"We'll have you ready," Sierra says.

I smile and keep going.

"You're doing great," she says, "getting stronger."

I pause between sets.

"Actually, I wonder if I should just ease up and forego this race," I say.

Sierra gives me a slow half nod.

"I mean, I *could* push it out to the fall."

She takes a couple of steps in my direction, looks at me, her kindness balanced by candor, and says, "I don't know how long you'll be able to run marathons, Allan. Let's try to get you ready for this one."

LATER

"How did it get so late so soon?" None other than Theodore Geisel, aka Dr. Seuss, gets credit for asking this question. It reminds me of similar questions and statements. *Where does the time go? Time is precious. You blink and it's over. The days are long but the years are short. Time flies. How did it get so late so soon?*

In graduate school, I became conscious of the fact that, in one sense, all of us have the same amount of time in a given day. We all have twenty-four hours to make use of, and we make choices on how we use our time that reflect necessity and need, but also desire and joy. On the other hand, those of us who live with more privilege, financial and otherwise, often have more free time at our disposal than those who live with less. Working two or three jobs leaves you with less time for other things than working one job typically does.

WATCHING THE TIME

Having Parkinson's tempts you to become a timekeeper if not a clock-watcher. You become more aware of time and you think about it more often than before. There is the time between visits with your neurologist, which comes with gauging your disease progression; and the time between your doses of medicine, which you learn to make precise in order to optimize your functioning. There is also the time you hope you have to keep work-ing, to stay active with your children or grandchildren, to live your life with time on your side. Of course, there is also the time you have wasted: on worry, anger, envy, and regret. In the words of the ancient philosopher, Seneca, "It's not that we have a short time to live, but that we waste a lot of it."[1] Parkinson's enhances this awareness, too. As Muhammad Ali, who also lived with Parkinson's, urged, "Don't count the days. Make the days count."[2]

1. Seneca, *On the Shortness of Life*, 1.
2. Ali, "21 of Muhammad Ali's Best Quotes."

Not long after Sierra's sobering reminder, former NBA icon Kobe Bryant died in a helicopter crash, along with his thirteen-year-old daughter, Gianna, and seven others. Bryant was just forty-one, and hitting his stride in life after basketball. Then, my close friend learned that his cancer was inoperable; and over 500 people have died from the coronavirus, with tens of thousands infected and no end in sight.

How did it get so late so soon?

It turns out that I might not get to run this marathon after all. Nagging injuries make it painful to push through the miles. My knee seems OK; my right foot, not so much. Plantar fasciitis? A stress fracture? My doctor will tell me in a couple of days, when I see her. Whatever happens, I will remain grateful for Sierra's gentle reminder of the importance of making the days count.

Every single one of them.

32

GOING PUBLIC

MY DECEPTION

About six weeks after my Parkinson's diagnosis, my cell phone rings and when I answer it my mother wastes no time before telling me why she has called.

"I just got a call from a doctor's office in Houston. They wanted to confirm an upcoming appointment with *Allan Cole*," she says.

"Hmm," I say, hoping to seem calm as my heart tries to leap out of my body.

"I thought it was strange, and I wanted to make sure you're OK," she says.

"Uh, I'm fine, Mom . . . but what exactly did they say?"

"They said they were calling to confirm an appointment with Allan Cole, and I told the woman who called she must be looking for a different Allan Cole [note that my father and I have the same name], as we live in North Carolina; then she apologized for having the wrong number, and that was it. I don't remember the doctor's name, or even if she said it, but they were in Houston, which seemed strange, and I started to worry that they might be calling for you."

"I'm sorry you were concerned, Mom, but I don't know anything about it . . . Occasionally, I get calls, too . . . from people looking for a different Allan Cole. Usually debt collectors. I guess there are a few of us out there."

My heart aches.

"I just wanted to make sure you're OK," Mom says.

I tell her not to worry, and, again, that I am fine. Then I change the subject.

As soon as I get off the phone with her, I dial the office of a neurologist I am scheduled to see in a few weeks, to investigate whether someone from his office has mistakenly called my parents' home, though this scenario makes no sense. When the receptionist answers, I tell her that I am calling to confirm my appointment, but also to make sure they have the correct phone number for me. She confirms the appointment and asks me my number, which matches what they have on file.

"And that's the only number you have for me, correct?"

"Yes, that's the only number we have," she says. "Would you like to provide an additional one?"

"No, thank you," I say.

And that was that.

To this day, I do not know whom my mother spoke with, what doctor's office called her, how they got my parents' phone number, or why they called.

I do know that I lied to my mother about my condition, and that doing so proved painful.

KEEPING IT CLOSE

Several people I know keep their Parkinson's diagnosis private. Perhaps a spouse, partner, children, or one or two close friends know they have Parkinson's, but no one else does. In some cases, it requires a great deal of effort to keep it this way as they camouflage or explain away their symptoms. I can relate to those who choose this path; I followed it myself for nearly a year after my own diagnosis.

There are good reasons to keep a diagnosis private. After all, Parkinson's comes with many misperceptions, naivety, as well as flat-out wrong assumptions about what it will mean for a person's future.

A few weeks after I shared my diagnosis publicly—which I did in an op-ed on health care reforms—I had lunch with a former colleague who compassionately told me how sorry he was to learn I have *Alzheimer's* disease. It was clearly a slip of the tongue and he blushed. He apologized profusely, turned even redder, and laughed with embarrassment before changing the subject. He knows the difference between Alzheimer's and

Parkinson's, but, as I would learn, not everyone does and there would be opportunities for education.

Even if they know the differences between these diseases, when people know we have Parkinson's they can begin to view us differently, even though they might not be aware of it. We can become objects of their pity, or they might feel less comfortable in our presence because they do not know what to say. Parkinson's can be a conversation stopper, no doubt.

Others' discomfort with our condition also may result in their becoming more distant, emotionally if not physically, such that we feel less included in their lives and lose access to them. In a similar vein, we may receive fewer invitations in both our social and professional circles. With respect to the latter, remember, too, that some of us who keep quiet about our Parkinson's are still working. We fear that supervisors or coworkers knowing of our condition will prompt them to assume we are less able to do our jobs, even if our performance has not changed, and even when given appropriate accommodations required by law.

I feared all of this and more; and, with one or two exceptions, *none* of it has happened.

PUTTING IT OUT THERE

On the other hand, living so cautiously, if not secretively, carries its own risks.

I felt disingenuous while carrying my secret, as if I was cheating on people I care about as well as being unfaithful to myself. I also felt a strong desire to use my situation for doing something constructive, such as raising awareness, providing education, and fundraising for Parkinson's organizations, as well as advocacy for more humane policies pertaining to health care and disability. I imagined feeling empowered by these efforts, buoyed by joining with others in solidarity, and, as a result, living with more purpose and hope.

However, doing any of this required being public with my disease, which I kept resisting.

As many secrets do, it weighed on me. A lot. Eventually, the secret wielded power that prevented me from living the kind of life I wanted to live.

THINGS TO CONSIDER

Few decisions feel more personal or crucial than deciding whether to disclose a serious medical condition. Many factors come into play when making this decision, and there is never a one-size-fits-all approach or outcome. Each of us must plot our own path.

Of course, the nature of having Parkinson's is such that, eventually, there comes a time when hiding it is no longer possible. Symptoms will have their say. Still, here are a few things to consider when discerning whether, when, and how to tell others about your condition.

What will you gain by being public?

Rather than focusing *first* on risks or potential losses, ask yourself what you expect to gain. What can you do once you are public that you cannot do now? Perhaps you will get more involved in Parkinson's-related activities or causes. Maybe you will become part of a support group or exercise community and enjoy their benefits. Perhaps you will reset personal priorities in ways that bring you added meaning and purpose, excitement and joy. Maybe you will feel less anxious, and more authentic and free, once you stop hiding or camouflaging your symptoms, or, as I did, lying about your status. As Toni Morrison put it in her book, *Song of Solomon*: "You wanna fly, you got to give up the shit that weighs you down."[1]

What will you risk losing or giving up?

Nevertheless, disclosure usually comes with losses, too; or at least with the risk of loss. I have already mentioned some of these potential losses, including a loss of status or standing, whether professionally or socially, as people's misassumptions and naivety about Parkinson's lead to treating you differently or in ways that hurt. Though relatively rare, I hope, some in our community report having experienced this kind of treatment. Either way, once others identify you as a person with Parkinson's, it is unlikely you will ever be able to live completely beyond that identity. You will give up your status as a healthy person. You might give up opportunities to advance in your career as well, or to change employers because you worry about the implications for health insurance.

If you are still working, have you consulted with an employment attorney?

Which brings me to a practical matter: I urge you to meet with an employment attorney prior to going public with your disease; in fact, it should

1. Morrison, *Song of Solomon*, 179.

be part of the discernment process. You will benefit from knowing your rights as well as your employer's responsibilities if you run into problematic responses. You want to make the most informed decisions you can with respect to living publicly with Parkinson's, including at work; the law is on your side with respect to your job, and knowing as much as possible about that can provide a measure of comfort and security.

NO REGRETS

I do not regret telling others about my having Parkinson's disease. I am fortunate to have a supportive spouse, family, friends, colleagues, and community, and their encouragement buoys me regularly and helps me integrate Parkinson's losses and gains in my life. And most of what I feared has not come to pass.

A part of me wishes I had shared my news even sooner.

It was a long, lonely, difficult first year of silence.

It feels much better not to live so weighed down.

And to tell my truth.

33

EMBRACING THE SUCK

COURAGE

You can feel the anticipation in the growing crowd. Students, faculty, staff, as well as people from Austin and beyond, gather in Gregory Gym on The University of Texas at Austin's campus. Nearly 4,000 of us have come to listen to Brené Brown talk about courageous leadership.

And more.

Trained as a social worker, she writes and speaks around the world to a variety of audiences: business leaders, elite athletes, the Army's Special Forces, and leading educators among them. She also speaks to regular folks, to all of us really, who seek to live less encumbered by fear and other detractors from a more authentic, courageous, and joy-filled life.

VULNERABILITY AND SHAME

Whatever the audience, Brené always talks about vulnerability and its constant hindrance, shame. Vulnerability means living with uncertainty, risk, and emotional exposure—all of which may be sources of courage. Shame, on the other hand, is the "intensely painful feeling or experience of believing that we are flawed and therefore unworthy of love and belonging—something we've experienced, done, or failed to do makes us unworthy of connection."[1] To think of it in slightly different terms, shame involves feeling overly exposed, and ties to concerns over our self-worth and falling short of what we perceive as others' expectations of us, which breeds fear. Too often, experiences of shame and related fear have a destructive effect on how we think, feel, relate, and, yes, lead; how we see the world and those in it, including ourselves.

Brené's genius is that she recognizes that most of us live with pervasive shame, which ultimately quells our courage and prevents the kind of vulnerability that offers more joy. She sees, too, that this bind we live in is self-inflicted, and we can learn to free ourselves by getting better at and more comfortable with, as she puts it, "showing up and being seen," authentically, for who we are. We find joy by shedding shame's armor, which we wear because we think it protects us, and instead "embracing the suck" of life's challenges that come our way, living with uncertainty, risk, and emotional exposure—that is, living with vulnerability—and striving for a more authentic and courageous life.

EXPOSURE

Less than two hours earlier, just a mile or so from campus, I sit with a group of friends for our own foray into living more vulnerably and with less armor. Two things brought us together last year, Parkinson's disease and our common connection to The University of Texas as professors and, in some cases, administrators. All of us are men, and everyone but me is retired; I am usually a "youngster" in most Parkinson's crowds. But that's just fine. I love being a part of this group, and I value these brilliant and wise souls mentoring me for the journey that lies ahead with the Parkinson's beast.

We meet at least once a month, at my friend Gary's house, and, get this, we talk about *ourselves*. I know . . . men don't usually talk about themselves, at least not in any vulnerable way. Instead, we talk about sports, politics, global events, work, and our families, but rarely about ourselves unless it has to do with an accomplishment or our success. As Frank McCourt put it, "You have to give yourself credit, [but] not too much because that would be bragging."[2]

---

1. Brown, "Shame v. Guilt."
2. McCourt, *Teacher Man*, 28.

SHOWING UP AND BEING SEEN

But not this group. What makes it special is that we have learned to remove some of our armor and to talk about ourselves; and about deeply personal things: physical and emotional challenges, our deepest fears, our longings, our regrets. It is a risky but safe space, a vulnerable space. It's one where tremors, stiffness, shuffling feet, masked faces, swallowing problems, slurred speech, flat affect, insomnia, REM sleep disorder, restless legs, incontinence, constipation, erectile dysfunction, hypersexuality, depression, anxiety, balance or gait problems, blood pressure issues, or having any other Parkinson blemish is OK.

We simply show up and allow ourselves to be seen.

We sit together, with less armor, sipping tea, coffee, wine, or water; eating snacks; longing for better days and yet grateful for what we still have; more exposed, yes, but with less fear; embracing the suck, together.

There is more freedom in that than I ever would have imagined possible three and a half years ago.

It all has something to do with what Brené Brown says: "We don't have to do all of it alone. We were never meant to."[3]

---

3. Brown, *Rising Strong*, 117.

34

PANDEMICS AND LONELINESS

QUIET

At 4 o'clock in the afternoon, I am the only one left in my area of the building. Classes cancelled, staff working from home, students enjoying an early spring break. Looking outside, a typically vibrant campus trafficked by the population of a midsized city feels listless.

The coronavirus has made its way to Austin.

Walking down the central hallway in my school's charming but old building, I hear only the HVAC system blowing; white noise, as it's called. The little voices normally echoing from the adjacent Child Development Center's playground are not there, nor are the typical conversations among students and faculty. Also missing are humming engines and squealing breaks of buses that pass by regularly beyond the front driveway.

What so many watched unfold from afar—first in China, then in Europe, and then on the left and right US coasts—has made its way here, to Austin and The University of Texas campus.

We knew it would happen but somehow temporarily reasoned it away.

ANXIETY

People get sick and die from this virus, especially those over sixty, but not exclusively so. Children and young adults can die, too, as can those with compromised health; and honestly, who cares about a person's age when that person is one you love?

This virus takes other tolls. People lose income, and with that the ability to feed their families, to pay their rent and other bills, and, for too many in our midst, to pay for the medicines and health care they depend on.

If you struggle before a pandemic hits . . .

The weight of all of this feels heavier than before; closer, too.

LONELINESS

"Social distancing" is the newly coined term. It began with prohibitions on shaking hands and hugging, and now requires not being within six feet of another person. It's the most effective means for slowing the infection rates, or "flattening the curve" of the disease, another new term for most of us outside epidemiology and health care circles.

In other words, the best thing we can do if we think we have been exposed to this devious little bastard—and who can really know—is to isolate ourselves from others, at least physically, and wait it out. For those coming in direct contact with someone infected, this means a two-week physical exile from everyone—family and friends, colleagues and neighbors, and anyone else with whom we typically share our lives.

I know, a little isolation might sound appealing on some level, but it is more challenging than it sounds and has a shadow side.

It heals us but dehumanizes us.

Human beings are social creatures. We gravitate toward other humans, naturally form emotional *and* physical bonds, and we plan and live our lives accordingly. What we do ties closely to those we do it with. What we find meaning in and what we enjoy, by and large, happens with trusted and valued others. Even among introverts like me!

Not only this, but when we face fear, worry, uncertainty, or other challenges, in most cases, most of the time, we reach out first to those we most value and love, *physically* as well as relationally, with words and gestures, yes, but also handshakes and hugs.

This hit me crossways today as I met with eleven trusted colleagues using Zoom. Gathered from twelve different places, we accomplished our goals; but it wasn't the same. In two weeks, we begin teaching our classes the same way.

We want to be in the presence of others, in an embodied way. It is essentially human.

I experienced this desire firsthand three and one-half years ago, when Parkinson's disease hit me crossways and became a part of my life. In an odd way, coronavirus feels like that. It is different, and the same. At least the loneliness part; and the self-isolation.

As Dorothy Day recognized, "We have all known the long loneliness and we have learned that the only solution is love and that love comes with community."[1]

Absent the physical presence of those most dear to us—family, friends, colleagues, students, neighbors; missing our *communities* in their fullest forms—we ache.

And hope.

1. Day, *The Long Loneliness*, 286.

35

THE BACK OF THE SANCTUARY

THE SANCTUARY

It is a Sunday morning, nearly a year since my diagnosis. Still living in the Parkinson's closet, I push through most days feeling afraid and alone. Even with my family and several friends a few feet away, today is no different.

I sit silently in the sanctuary.

My wife and our daughters and I gravitated here a few months ago. This small community of people from nearly every continent and with nearly every skin tone offers open hearts and shares open minds. This church's racial and ethnic diversity attracts us, as do its commitments to social, economic, and environmental justice.

What most draws us is its conscience.

These folks extend hospitality to the poor, homeless, pilgrim, and stranger. Fortunately, they also welcome those trying to figure some things out.

THE JOURNEY

Sitting at the back of the sanctuary, as I typically do, I think about how I got here.

A distant cousin jarred my more or less placid religious quest when I was in the sixth grade. Embracing a fundamentalist flavor of Christianity, he scared the shit out of me with his talk of the Antichrist and pending doomsday scenarios, things like the rapture and Apocalypse, which I'd never heard of before but which he swore were clearly "prophesied" in the Bible. I was an Episcopalian, after all; and while I knew Rites I and II of the Holy Eucharist by heart, I had no clue what the Bible said or did not say.

I had to ask what *prophesied* meant.

Other than for that period, however, I mostly found comfort in my family's religion and in church. There, I learned stories about Jesus, who treated people with compassion and healed them. I spent time with flawed human beings aiming to follow his example and latch on to his hope. Churches were enchanted places that housed mystery and intrigue. They made me tingle and feel warm. I loved their smells and their people. In church, I experienced what the psychologist Erik H. Erikson called a sense of at-home-ness in the world.

Sometimes, I still do.

THE MOSAIC

Back to the congregation gathered here: they come with authenticity and vulnerability, with compassion and generosity. They come as those who struggle, hurt, and hope. Collectively, they come to learn about and live out the values of Jesus of Nazareth.

He taught and modeled these values, saying, "Blessed are the peacemakers" (Matthew 5:9); "Whoever has two coats must share with anyone who has none; and whoever has food must do likewise" (Luke 3:11); and "you shall love your neighbor as yourself" (Matthew 22:39).

The clear day's sun shines through the mosaic of stained glass that surrounds the triangular chancel. At certain moments, its colors pop out as if hoping to land in worshipers' laps. A woman in her late twenties plays "Morning Has Broken" beautifully on her violin.

From the back of the sanctuary, I take all of this in.

My mind drifts to experiences of the past year: a faint tremor in my left index finger, an initial misdiagnosis, multiple exams, a brain scan, sleepless nights, worries, loneliness, and tears. Staring at the stained glass, I consider my mosaic of beliefs: about justice and mercy; fairness and equity; pain and comfort; meaning and purpose; despair and hope.

I also consider if I any longer sense a presence of the divine, whether in churches or in my life.

Wondering what life might require in the years to come, I look to my right, where Holly, Meredith, and Tracey sit, and fight back tears as my daughters draw in their sketchbooks.

A guitarist plays another musical piece while a trio sings along.

THE PILGRIMS

I look around the room, taking account of others who have come to church that day. Most are members who attend weekly. Many face the tensions of living a burdened and faithful life.

There is Caleb, a sweet, interesting, and bright twelve-year-old boy with autism. He works valiantly each day to go to school, to interact peaceably with others, and to be a typical kid. Once, he invited Tracey over for dinner and the rest of us got to join her. His remarkable parents seated beside him, Sarah and Sam, tirelessly advocate for Caleb, model pure vulnerability coupled with exquisite courage and grace, and never cease cheering him on. All of us do.

There is also Ruth, an older woman with a gentle disposition and astute mind whose medical condition has her confined to a wheelchair, and for whom living alone gets more and more challenging. She sits next to Nancy, who faithfully and tenderly cares for her friend, and whose political positions impress me.

Julio and Astrid are there as well. They will marry in a little over a year, and I think of Julio's longtime separation from his family because of immigration concerns. His family cannot get back into the US from their native Mexico, in spite of having lived here for many years.

Then, I see Leslie, who lives courageously, with dignity, and at enviable peace with advancing breast cancer that has metastasized. Her contagious, resolute smile simultaneously heartens and convicts me. Months later, she will be in hospice care.

I also see Jose, a kind and brawny man in his late thirties, surrounded by his lovely parents as well as by his siblings, nieces, and nephews. All of them, along with the larger church community, have prayed for Jose while he sought sobriety and spent nearly a decade in prison. Recently released, he hopes to get his life back on track.

Then I flash back to Kate, a middle-aged woman who lives on the streets. She wandered into the church a couple of weeks earlier and we met in front of the large coffee urn. Her clean white coffee cup stood in stark contrast to her dirty fingernails and the dinge of homelessness that covered her. She heard voices and seemed scared and suspicious. Like many of us, she was there looking for connection, significance, and hope.

THE SACRED

Life is not easy.

We get sick, lose those we love, struggle for meaning, seek after peace, and clamor for justice. These days, we also worry about pandemics and crushing need on a global scale. We experience a lot of adversity.

Surrounded by all of this, and more, we desire to have a place in communities that value us, reassure us, companion us, and urge us on. Perhaps as we also long for clues of a divine presence in our lives.

If not now, eventually. It has always been this way. It is the human condition.

I have spent much of my life looking for answers to the big life questions, religious and otherwise. For decades I searched mostly in books, whether when reading them or writing them, and by sorting through the ideas and insights of the sages.

Now, I'm more apt to look for answers, or at least possibilities, in people and relationships, in shared struggles as well as joys, in those who stand in solidarity against any form of injustice and dedicate themselves to creating something better.

Really, I hone in on where I see efforts within a community to love, to be loved, and, as the Bible says, "to share one another's burdens" (Galatians 6:2).

You can learn a lot sitting in the back of a sanctuary.

Sometimes, you can even catch a glimpse of the divine.

36

LIFE BY THE HOUR

THE ZOOMING HOUR

Sometimes, life dishes out disappointment. Something happens that does not match our hopes or expectations.

Like when Audrey recently defended her dissertation, the last requirement for completing her PhD program in social work at The University of Texas at Austin.

It is late morning when eight of us meet online. Zooming in from different locations around Austin, all sheltered in place, we have anticipated this joyous occasion—some for weeks, others for months and even years. Nevertheless, with COVID-19 leaving its mark, it is not as we had hoped or expected.

Viewing one another through webcams, we don headsets and microphones, looking like participants on *Hollywood Squares* or characters on *The Brady Bunch* crossed with airline pilots or radio DJs.

After a few exchanges of pleasantries, Audrey's dissertation defense begins. Leading us through her project, answering our questions, demonstrating her expertise, she flourishes, as she has throughout her program. It is a memorable day, the culmination of rigorous doctoral studies four years in the making.

Our gathering certainly feels joyful and celebrative, but also a tad disappointing—*bittersweet*.

Why? Because we cannot meet in person and exchange celebratory handshakes and hugs; and Audrey will not have a graduation ceremony this spring, when her family and friends and the larger community would recognize her accomplishment; and we are living in a liminal space, anxious and unsettled, not knowing what the next days, weeks, or months will bring.

It feels like we are shortchanging her as COVID-19 leaves its mark.

THE LONGING HOUR

I think back to something my friend Elizabeth told me recently. Her friend is distraught over not being able to visit the nursing home where her elderly mother is cared for. This parent lives with dementia, and her daughter worries that she will not understand the circumstances and will assume she has been abandoned.

I also hark back to when Tracey told me that women giving birth in hospitals are having to do so without their birth partners by their sides—all part of social distancing and other pandemic safety measures. Do these mothers and their partners feel abandoned or shortchanged, too?

I wonder as well about other significant occasions we will lose—weddings, bat mitzvahs, birthday parties, book clubs, ball games, dance recitals—and the connections we will miss and the life experiences we will forego as we socially distance ourselves, flatten the curve of exposure to this virus, and, we hope, inch ourselves back to some measure of normalcy.

THE LIVING HOUR

As I reflect on all of this, and as I sit with the pain it causes, I remember something I learned from Robert Frost many years ago, when I was a student myself. He said, "In three words I can sum up everything I've learned about life: it goes on."[1]

When our hopes and expectations go unfulfilled . . . life goes on.

Which brings me to those of us who live with Parkinson's disease. We know something about hopes and expectations going unfulfilled. These disappointments come by way of physical challenges, emotional pain,

1. Josephs, "Robert Frost's Secret."

relational renegotiations, professional pivots, and social distancing of another sort.

Perhaps we are left feeling shortchanged if not abandoned.

But should we expect it to be otherwise?

A line in Margaret Mitchell's classic novel *Gone with the Wind* says, "Life's under no obligation to give us what we expect."[2]

In other words, life sometimes disappoints.

But it also satisfies, even amid its disappointments. This we cannot forget.

Babies still come into the world; the frail elderly still get cared for; and hard-working students still graduate and prosper. Not only this, but those of us with Parkinson's still love, work, laugh, cry, contribute, guide, share, nurture, embrace, give thanks, and hope.

Accordingly, *life* goes on.

2. Mitchell, *Gone with the Wind*, 1291.

37

A LETTER TO MY DAUGHTER
ON DETERMINATION

April 5, 2020

Dear Holly,

I often think back to that spring day in 2017, when you were nine and I had not yet told you about my having Parkinson's disease; hardly anyone knew. I had not yet mustered up the courage to share it. I was afraid of what life could be like once people knew. How would they see me? Would they think I was too sick to keep doing things together? Honestly, in those first months after my diagnosis, I was not sure how I would keep going.

But I knew I had to figure it out.

Then, one Saturday afternoon, as I sat in our living room reading, you opened the front door, called for me, and said, "I think I'm ready, Daddy."

Wearing your new purple leotard with pink and white accents, you gestured for me to follow you outside, which I did. When you turned around, I noticed your long, curly hair pulled back in a tight ponytail. It was held by a color-coordinated scrunchie that I'm sure you had carefully chosen. You always take your time choosing what you put in your hair.

I remember how strong and poised you looked.

As a dedicated gymnast, you spent several hours each week in our front yard working on your tumbling, which built on the formal practice you got at your gymnastics school. You had your mind set on learning a new skill, a round off back handspring that ends with a back tuck; what I called your back flip. You worked hard to learn it. Almost every day.

I watched you practice every chance I could. Sometimes, I watched from our yard, cheering you on as you made attempt after attempt. Other times, I peered stealthily through our living room bay window. You kept getting better at your tumbling routines; and you kept adding new elements. You also got more confident—I could see it in your face.

When you began learning to tumble, you could barely flip your body and I held my breath each time you took off running across the front yard. I could hear the sound of your petite muscular frame whiz by, followed by several determined grunts.

After days of trying, when you finally did a full flip, you landed like a frog, with your butt on the ground and your legs folded up under you. Actually, you landed this way dozens of times over the course of several more days of hard work. Still, you kept at it, day after day, week after week: whizzing by, grunting, flying through the air. Eventually, you went from landing like a frog to landing more like a filly, trying to steady your legs under you without falling over.

Then, one Saturday afternoon, it was time.

I can still picture it, as if it is happening at this moment.

With a running start, you speed cross our front yard. Lunging forward into a round off, then into a back handspring, and then into a back tuck, your little body folds up with purpose. Then, in an instant, you unwind and land with your legs fully extended, like a confident eagle reaching out before a perch. You quickly arch your back and your arms shoot high in the air. Your two giant dimples flank your gaping smile. As they say in gymnastics, you stick the landing!

I will always remember this day.

I mention it because three years later I have come to realize that my living with Parkinson's is a lot like you learning to do that back handspring with a back tuck. What I mean is that for me to live well with Parkinson's I have to work at it. I have to push through harder days, like when my legs feel like a frog's or a filly's, or when my body does not work as it used to, as I want it to. Just as you did, I have to keep challenging myself to stick with it, to be persistent.

I need to get out of bed in the morning, take my medicine, eat a good breakfast, run or go to the gym, get myself to work, and aim to be productive. I need to get adequate sleep, try to reduce stress, eat healthy food, and stay connected to the people I care about and who care about me—Mom, you and Meredith, Grams and Papa, Nonni, Aunt Marie, Tom and my other friends, our neighbors, and my colleagues at UT.

Really important too, I stay in close contact with other people who live with Parkinson's: Ethan, Allie, Bret, Bill, Jimmy, Heather, Chris, and lots of others—you know most of them. We support one another in ways that I guess can only happen if you have Parkinson's and know what it is like to have to work at managing it.

But I have to do some other things, too—and these are things I learned from watching you. I have to keep a positive attitude, and tolerate my frustrations, and learn from disappointing experiences or setbacks.

After all, who sticks every landing?

Most important, I have trust not only that I can live well with this illness, but I can keep getting better at it.

I promise I will keep working hard to do just that.

Thank you for teaching me how.

Love,
Daddy
P.S. Have you finished your homework?

38

TIRES AND TESTS

———————

The four of us have just left Frankie's house and gotten on Mo Pac Expressway when we hear it: *thump, thump, thump, thump, thump, thump, thump* . . . If you have ever heard this sound, then you know immediately what it is.

Frankie is my daughter Meredith's closest friend and today is her fourteenth birthday. Since COVID-19 and physical distancing have nixed any party, we decide to ride by Frankie's house and sing "Happy Birthday" to her and her family—us in the car at the curb, with them standing on their front lawn. After being "quarantined" for nearly three weeks and counting, this drive-by serenade should give us all a little boost. I hope Frankie feels celebrated.

After slowly exiting Mo Pac and parking the car on a neighborhood side street, I lift up the hatchback, locate the spare tire, jack, and other tools I will need, and get to work. My wife Tracey, our girls, and one of our dogs, Hank, sit on the curb and offer commentary on the scene. A man about my age rides by on a fancy bicycle and asks, "Are y'all OK?" After Tracey assures him that we are, he waves and pedals by while keeping six to eight feet away.

I literally have not changed a flat tire in decades. When Tracey or I have a flat, we just call AAA and they come fix it. It is the best deal you can get for $56 a year. Still, we are in the middle of a pandemic; and who knows whether AAA can even send someone to help; and we need to get our other daughter Holly home for her dance class via Zoom; and Meredith has homework . . . and, well, I have Parkinson's disease . . .

So I am changing that fucking tire!

Slightly loosening the lug nuts, I place the jack in the appropriate place on the car's frame, just in front of the rear wheel well. Then, with my left arm mildly shaking as I reach for the handle, I slowly turn it and the car begins to lift.

One of the most common Parkinson's symptoms is hand tremors, especially when the hands are at rest. I do not have much of that. What I do have is a stiff left arm, wrist, and hand; and when they become fatigued—like when carrying something heavy, such as a tire; or when gripping something tightly for several seconds, such as a tire iron; or when loosening lug nuts or turning a jack handle—they can start to shake a little and hurt. Couple this shaking with the constant lack of dexterity in my left hand, and it leaves a lot to be desired.

Did I mention that I am left-handed?

This is my life with Parkinson's.

So far, it is mostly little things that are getting harder. Writing and typing, buttoning a shirt and shaving, gripping a pair of pliers, threading lug nuts properly in order to tighten them back up. Using a screwdriver. And please, don't ask me to thread a needle!

Here's the thing: being able to do the little things, even when I am shaky at it, helps me believe I'll be able to do the bigger things longer, and not have to call on somebody to do these bigger things for me.

I tighten the last lug nut holding the spare tire in place. In all, it takes about forty-five minutes, and Holly will make her dance class. As I wipe the sweat from my forehead and pack up my tools, I think back to one day earlier, when Meredith reminded me that she will be driving in two years. When she mentioned this, I told her that in order to drive, and even before she takes the test for her license, she has to show me she can change a flat tire. "You can't always depend on AAA," I said, "and it's a life skill everyone should have."

Who knew that less than twenty-four hours later she would have a front row seat watching her dad change a tire?

As part of his own test?

39

DRIVE, DIGNITY, AND DREAMS

Still Got It, declares the large orange font placed off to the side of his left shoulder. A handsome and fit older man, he has pulled a full bag of groceries from the back of his SUV, with his taut chest, thick neck, and right arm semi-flexed. If there were still any doubt, his sculpted calves have "athlete" written all over them. He smiles in an effortful Parkinson's way.

Above his shoulder it reads, *Still got drive. Still got dignity. Still got dreams.*

In smaller text, just below the knees, he introduces himself and shares the remainder of his message: "My name is Phil, and support is there for us if we need it."

Hi, Phil, I say to myself, *I am all for support, but let's talk.*

Turns out it is an ad for Rytary, an extended release form of carbidopa/levodopa, the gold standard of Parkinson's treatment and a medication that I, and millions of others with Parkinson's, take. Taking it can allow you to move, literally, when Parkinson's makes you feel like a stone statue; and it gives you an energy boost when fatigue grips every cell in your body. I am grateful for this medicine.

Nevertheless, *Still Got It* irritates me. It irritates me because it's linked to Phil's drive, dignity, and dreams—things that lie at the heart of being human, whether you live with an illness or not. Do those at Impax Laboratories, the makers of Rytary, believe that as Parkinson's progresses and takes our ability for movement, it also takes our determination, self-respect, and hopes for the future? Does Phil believe this? If so, does he see Rytary as the solution?

I am learning that too often those living with illness, including my brothers and sisters who have Parkinson's, succumb to the assumptions, descriptions, prescriptions, and expectations of the healthy. We defer our "insider" perspectives on illness to those of "outsiders," meaning those who are *not yet* ill.

Philosopher Havi Carel, who lives with her own serious illness, a chronic pulmonary condition, observes that, "Being a good ill person, a good patient, is conforming to the expectations of the healthy, not to be offended or polluted by your illness. When you begin to get praise for your behavior, then you know you have achieved the status of a conformist. An ill conformist conforming to the demands of the healthy majority, who cannot, will not, wills not to see the fate that awaits us all."[1]

Impax Laboratories places the norms and expectations of the healthy front and center in its ad. Calling on us to conform.

Here is what I want to say to Impax Laboratories, and especially to Phil.

Phil, you look like you are faring well with Parkinson's, and that in itself inspires me. But here's what I want you to know about me.

I have to work harder to move, and to sleep, and to do other things I once took for granted. But my dreams have never been more vivid or clear: to live a meaningful life; to make contributions to the common good; to be a good husband, dad, son, colleague, and citizen; to dance with my daughters at their weddings. And while I have the same types of insecurities that every human being has, including some tied to having Parkinson's, I've never felt more centered in who I am or more accepting of myself, so my dignity is intact. And, you think Parkinson's has taken my drive? Well, as my feet hit the floor each morning, and I power on my laptop to start a day of writing, and I lace up my shoes to go for run, and I get on my bike to ride with my daughters, and I say "Good morning" to a class of social work students at The University of Texas at Austin—I'm as driven as ever to live a full, purposeful, productive, generous, compassionate, and meaningful life.

Please tell Impax Laboratories to tell their ad agency all of that.

One more thing, Phil, and please share this, too.

---

1. Havi Carel, *Illness*, 67. Carel is paraphrasing the insights of sociologist Irving Goffman.

Never confuse health, ability, or functioning with determination, self-worth, or aspirations. Never mistake what we can or cannot do for who we are. Never allow illness take hold of your humanity. Because when you can no longer drive that SUV, or lift those groceries, or inhabit that chiseled body, you'll still be you. You'll still have value. You'll still be human.

Maybe more human than ever.

It's time for my next dose of Rytary.

40

A NEW NORMAL?

MASKS

After I park, a petite, middle-aged woman quickly approaches my car, her hands protected by blue latex gloves, her olive-colored face covered by a floral-patterned homemade mask. It reminds me of the heather green one I wear each time I leave my house. As she gets closer, I see her large, kind, and friendly brown eyes peering above white piping. They belie the severe social measures the pandemic has induced.

I think of the Billy Idol song "Eyes Without a Face."

Best Buy has their merchandise pick-up process down to a science. You pull into a designated area, park, pull up their app, click on the "I'm at the store" button, and give a description of your car. Soon thereafter, an associate comes out, opens your back door or reaches into an open window, trunk, or hatchback, and places your order in your car. How much easier could it get?

On the one hand, all of us have come for good reasons. The Best Buy employees are earning a living. I am purchasing a new router so that my family and I can Zoom—that is, use videoconferencing for work, school, and our social lives. We are simply doing life differently, these days, functioning in a new mode, adapting to what too many people describe as the "new normal."

On the other hand, I feel the weight of a socially distant and faceless world.

FACES

As it turns out, seeing faces matters. A lot. The French philosopher Emmanuel Levinas points us to why this is so. He identifies the unique power of the human face to make claims on us and orient us in the world: "[T]he face speaks to me and thereby invites me to a relation," and "it [is] a source from which all meaning appears."[1] More than this, face-to-face encounters obligate us to one another, meaning that with our faces we make moral and ethical claims on each other that are uniquely human. As Levinas puts it, "[T]he Other faces me and puts me in question and obliges me"[2] and "In front of the face, I always demand more of myself."[3] Face-to-face encounters change us and humanize us precisely because they obligate us to one another. The faces of others call on us to become the best version of human we can become.

In 2010, the contemporary performance artist Marina Abramovic held an exhibition in the New York Museum of Modern Art. Titled "The Artist is Present," she sat silently across a small table from strangers, one person at a time, as they each looked directly into one another's eyes.[4] This continued for nearly 747 hours across six weeks. Having sat across from over 1,500 people, Abramovic says it changed her forever: "completely— every possible element, every physical emotion." She says, "This enormous need of humans to actually have contact, how we are so alienated from each other, how society makes us really distant. We are texting each other messages without seeing each other . . . so many stories of loneliness. What's happening here? I'm looking at you."[5]

Whether belonging to a loved one, neighbor, friend, colleague, student, Best Buy associate, or stranger, a face reminds us of our common humanity. Constantly concealing our faces protects our health, but also makes it harder to see each other, harder to recognize humanity, in others and in ourselves.

1. Levinas, *Totality and Infinity*, 198, 297.
2. Levinas, *Totality and Infinity*, 207.
3. Levinas, "Signature."
4. Dwyer, "Confronting a Stranger."
5. Zec, dir., *Marina Abramovic*.

ZOOM

Which brings me back to Zoom.

For six weeks and counting, Zoom gets me to work and my kids to school, piano lessons, and dance classes. Zoom takes my family to doctor's appointments, and to virtual hangouts and happy hours with friends, whether in town or across the country. Feeling Zoomed-out on many days, I have wondered if we could all use a collective Zoomectomy!

Then, I remember.

When we Zoom, I get to see your face.

41

LET TOMORROW COME TOMORROW

YESTERDAY

It's now early in 2017, a few months after my Parkinson's diagnosis, and I keep trying to *learn* my way out of the illness. I have never had difficulty with living in my head.

I open my laptop and begin researching. The clock on the mantel tells me it's 5 AM. Some mornings I begin even earlier.

Pointing and clicking my way through websites and sifting through articles, I learn about the latest Parkinson's treatments, clinical trials, and groundbreaking research. I scroll through the list of the Parkinson's Foundation's Centers of Excellence, which distinguishes top-flight treatment centers across the world. I search out Parkinson's organizations, support groups, and ways to get involved . . . as soon as I tell people I have this illness.

In the meantime, as we do most mornings, Google and I search for reasons to hope.

We also meet most nights after my wife and children go to bed. As night glides into morning, I consume dozens of articles, books, and videos. Since my diagnosis remains a secret from everyone but my wife, Tracey, it feels like I am sneaking around to watch Parkinson's porn.

With certain videos, I plot out potential timelines for disease progression, noting how people appear to fare across a span of years. "Look at Michael J. Fox back in 1997," I say to Tracey one morning as I play the video from our kitchen's island, "and look at him now. After over twenty years with it, he still looks good; and he's working!"

I hone in on these videos like a scientist looking through a microscope in search of a breakthrough.

TODAY

Three years later, my colleague and I sit across from one another in my campus office sipping coffee. With midsemester demands pressing down on us, it's been weeks since we've spoken face to face.

Eventually, our conversation turns to my health. I never mind when it does, when someone asks how I am doing, though most who ask seem to feel awkward about it. Their "Do-you-mind-if-I-ask-about" type of introductory clause gives them away.

I understand the discomfort; it can be difficult to talk about illness. We assume, often mistakenly, that persons who live with illness could not be happy or content and that asking about their condition will only remind them of their pain.

For some of us, however, speaking about our illness brings meaning to the experience and disarms it; its powerful grip softens, if only a bit. It's enough to help.

After spending nearly a year in the Parkinson's closet, I decided that my attempts to make sense of this illness required speaking about it publicly, and with transparency and candor. I sometimes tell Tracey that I fear one day waking up and thinking, "Oh shit, what have I done? I shared too much!" But I'm willing to take this approach because the benefits are greater than the risk. Others may need to take a different, perhaps more private path, and I honor them and their choices.

On this occasion with my colleague, after a few brief exchanges, he asks, "What has changed since you were diagnosed? I mean, what is different now?"

It's a reasonable question when one lives with a progressive disease.

I tell him my symptoms remain manageable and are still only mildly disruptive, but I know this will change over time. I mention that my biggest problem right now is difficulty sleeping, a side effect of medication more than anything, and that I'm getting on average four hours each night and I'm trying to figure out a solution.

"That must be tough," he says.

"It's an acquired taste," I say.

He chuckles.

"What's changed, honestly, is I'm no longer consumed with how quickly this will progress, and with what life will be like five, ten, or fifteen years from now," I say.

He nods.

"I think about it, of course, but not like I used to. Instead, I really try to live in the moment, to live for today, to not miss seeing the beauty, love, meaning, joy, excitement, and opportunity that's right in front of me because my eyes are continuously peering over the horizon."

"What led to this new perspective?" he asks.

"I discovered how much time and energy I was spending on trying to figure out something for which there is no answer. Everything I read confirmed what my doctors told me, that you can't predict how Parkinson's will progress; its pace and severity are different for everyone."

He nods again.

"So I decided to put that time and energy into what I have today, what's life-giving, and beautiful, and true. A lot of this is fleeting, too, just like health, and I don't want to miss enjoying it all, as much as I can."

"That makes a lot of sense to me. I'm happy to hear you're in a better place with all of this," he says.

TOMORROW

I glance over my colleague's shoulder and see the rows of books that line my office bookshelves. These books tell a decades-long story of intellectual and existential questions and pursuits. I notice the bright red spine of Wendell Berry's *What Are People For?*—one of his many volumes of essays, its cover worn from so much use.

Remembering a Berry line, I quote it to my colleague: "Let tomorrow come tomorrow. Not by your will is the house carried through the night."[1]

Which is one way of saying that these days I work less at learning my way out of Parkinson's.

1. Berry, *What Are People For?*, 13.

42

WHY I PREFER ILLNESS TO DISEASE

WHAT DO YOU SEE?

About a year after my diagnosis with Parkinson's disease, I discovered the work of the British philosopher Havi Carel, who lives with a chronic and progressive lung condition, and who points out the importance of distinguishing *illness* from *disease*.

When we focus on disease, we tend to look at a person *objectively*, at a distance, and primarily in terms of the physical body and its dysfunction.[1] We hone in on what is wrong with hearts, or lungs, or brains, with vital organs and systems, and we linger on how medicine may help them work better and more efficiently.

Contrast this view with a focus on *illness*, which attends to the subjective, *so what*, questions of disease.[2] As Carel notes, "Illness is the *experience* of disease, the 'what it is like' qualitative dimension as it is experienced and made meaningful by the ill person."[3] In practical terms, viewing Parkinson's principally as an *illness* helps me hone in on the colors and contours of what my life is like, day to day, moment to moment.

The objective body and facts of disease certainly have their place in medicine. Like when I got a DaTscan to confirm a Parkinson's diagnosis.

1. Carel, *Phenomenology*, 15.
2. Carel, *Phenomenology*, 46.
3. Carel, *Phenomenology*, 17.

DISEASE

The barely lit room looks as cold as it feels. I lie down on a hard table that becomes the bottom half of a tube that covers most of my head and shoulders. About fifteen feet away, a technician who greeted me as I entered the room sits at a small control board. I can barely see his face as he explains the DaTscan procedure; neurologists sometimes order this scan as a way to help confirm a Parkinson's diagnosis. It is difficult to hear him due to the hum of a fan blowing fresh air, presumably to keep the imaging equipment cool. His shadowy silhouette, whose every third or fourth word I understand, reminds me of a Peanuts character: *blah, blah, imaging, blah, blah, blah, dopamine receptors, blah, blah, blah, blah, relax . . .*

He tells me what I already know. After reading about DaTscans, I have learned that this procedure provides an image of dopamine transporter activity in the brain. Particular patterns of activity are indicative of Parkinson's.

"Any questions?" he says.

"How long does my head have to stay clamped in this position?" I say.

"Usually it's about forty-five minutes," he says, pushing a few additional buttons.

He pauses.

"Any more questions?"

"This isn't your first rodeo, is it?" I say.

Silence.

"OK, here we go," he says.

The scan starts, and for what seems like an hour the camera tube moves around my head in strange patterns. A geary whine joins the white noise of the cooling fan. I have goose bumps on my skin.

Finally, the camera stops moving and the whine quiets so that only the sound of the fan remains. The room lightens and peripherally I see the tech approaching the table where I lay. My scalp burns, my head throbs. I am still woozy from a sedative a nurse gave me earlier, and the tech helps me stand and walks me back to the same room I was in earlier, where I lie down with a thin blanket, hoping to get warm.

Half an hour later, the same tech returns to walk me outside to the parking lot, where Tracey is waiting for me. When I get to the car's passenger door, the tech opens it, looks at me, and says, "Good luck."

This is what it is like to have someone see and treat your *disease*.

Don't get me wrong, I care about dopamine transporter activity; but only *because* a lack of it makes me feel poorly or prevents me from doing certain things I value. Otherwise, who thinks about how much dopamine activity you have going on in your brain?

But I care about other things, too, like when I'm seen as a whole person in relation to a disease that has come into my life. I want my doctor to attend to my illness, not just my disease.

ILLNESS

A week after my scan, Tracey and I walk into my neurologist's office together, just as he had asked us to do. This place looks different from when I first saw it: a little brighter and warmer, smaller and less like a maze. A friendly receptionist immediately invites us back to the same exam room where my life changed just four weeks earlier. We take a seat in chairs next to the small desk where I first showed Dr. T my labored handwriting. He is the one who ordered my DaTscan.

After only a minute or two, Dr. T enters the room wearing a colorful bow tie, wire-rimmed glasses, and a burnt orange lanyard with The University of Texas written on it that holds his St. David's Medical Center ID badge. He says "good morning" as I stand up, and we shake hands. He also extends his hand to Tracey and introduces himself to her.

"How are you two doing?" he asks.

"I think we're OK," I say. "Taking one day at a time . . . learning how to live with *the new family member.*"

He had offered this image of "the new family member who will always live with you" to describe Parkinson's.

He flashes a compassionate smile.

He then asks about my symptoms and how I am doing with the Azilect, the medicine he'd given me. I tell him I seem to be tolerating it just fine and that I think it's helping with the stiffness.

He nods.

"Well, I suspect you have some questions," he says.

I pull out an index card with questions I have prepared, and for nearly thirty minutes, I ask him about Parkinson's disease. I want to hear about the rate of disease progression and the different kinds of medicine he envisions me taking. I also ask him about resources for support in the Austin community. Of course, I have already researched all of these questions, but I am entrusting my neurological life to this man. I need him to weigh in.

I need him to invest, too.

He restates being confident about the disease progressing slowly, and when I ask about "falling off a cliff" with the disease, meaning I want to know if it will progress slowly with subtle changes for a period, but then accelerate and push me into a rapid decline, he assures me it will not. "It doesn't work that way. There are never any 100 percent guarantees, of course, but I think you're going to do well for a long time."

Tracey smiles, and places her hand on my back.

"I think so, too," she says.

He then shares his thinking about medications, including drugs that stimulate dopamine receptors (agonists) and replace depleted dopamine (carbidopa and levodopa) in your brain, and he touches briefly on a surgical procedure called Deep Brain Stimulation, or DBS. It is remarkably effective at relieving symptoms and its technology is getting better all the time; but DBS tends to be what you opt for when medicines become less effective. He also mentions two local organizations for which he has a high regard, Capital Area Parkinson's Society and Power for Parkinson's, which provides free exercise classes, and he encourages me to explore their offerings.

I tell him I will.

Seeing that I have no other questions, he looks over at Tracey.

"What questions do you have?"

She looks at me.

"He thinks I'm in denial, but, like you, I really believe he's going to do well. He's a fighter, and a good patient."

I put my arm around her.

"Just take good care of him. We need him." Her voice cracks slightly.

Dr. T flashes another kind smile.

"I will. He's going to do well."

Tracey pulls a bag of cookies from her purse and gives them to him— her chocolate biscotti. She is a professional baker.

"You want to make *sure* he's taken good care of," he says.

"You've got that right!" she says.

We say our goodbyes and leave his office.

Driving home, our new family member seems a little less intrusive, and I feel a little more human.

Like I have been seen.

43

A TIME TO TALK

When a friend calls to me from the road
And slows his horse to a meaningful walk,
I don't stand still and look around
On all the hills I haven't hoed,
And shout from where I am, "What is it?"
No, not as there is time to talk.
I thrust my hoe into the mellow ground,
Blade-end up and five feet tall,
And plod: I go up to the stone wall
For a friendly visit.

—Robert Frost, "A Time to Talk"[1]

ZOOMING

The laughter begins almost immediately, as one of us quips about needing a pandemic haircut and another about needing hair. Banter about being in and out of shape follows, and then comes mention of hand tremors, dyskinesia, insomnia, and other self-deprecating talk. Seven middle-aged men, all in our forties and fifties and sharing the moniker of young-onset Parkinson's disease, are Zooming on a Thursday night.

---

1. Frost, "A Time to Talk."

Bret is in New York, Chris in Connecticut, Ethan in DC, Bill and Jimmy in Chicago, I'm in Austin, and Jonathan, our Canadian friend, is in Vancouver, British Columbia. Brought together three years ago by illness, The Michael J. Fox Foundation for Parkinson's Research (MJFF), and a mutual interest in running marathons, now we live united in friendship, and in our desire to lead active and meaningful lives in spite of the Parkinson's beast.

We should have gathered in April in New York, an annual affair, in order to celebrate another year of work on behalf of MJFF. But COVID-19 put the skids on that plan. Missing these guys, I put together a Zoom call so we could connect, act less maturely or seriously for an hour or so, and catch up on one another's active, interesting, and Parkinson's-laden lives.

RECOLLECTING

Looking back three years, I met Bret and Jimmy first. Several months after my diagnosis, and still enduring anxiety-laced days and sleepless nights while tucked deep in the back of my Parkinson's closet, I reached out first to Bret and then to Jimmy, both of whom I found online due to their advocacy and efforts to raise awareness of Parkinson's.

I reached out to them because I needed to hope. I had to hear that I could still be the father I wanted to be, that the career I loved could continue far into the future, that I could find ways to contribute, encourage, raise awareness, and educate—to do some good with something so shitty. I needed to believe that I would be OK; and that my family would be OK; and that life could still be good and even joyful again.

Putting it another way, I reached out to Bret and Jimmy because I was suffering in silence and secrecy, and I needed what Emerson describes as, "a person with whom I may be sincere. Before [whom] I may think aloud."[2]

Bret and Jimmy allowed me to do both. This will come as no surprise to those who know them.

Shortly thereafter, I met the rest of this Zoom crew. I first spoke to Bill as he prepared to walk across the United States, from Georgia to California, which he accomplished in 2018; and shortly after that, I met Chris, Ethan, and Jonathan at a MJFF event, and we quickly became friends.

All of them generous souls, they have made my first miles down the Parkinson's road less lonely, more hopeful, and certainly more fun than I

2. Emerson, "Friendship," 119.

ever would have imagined possible when my neurologist's words stopped me in my tracks: "I think you're in the early stages of Parkinson's disease."

Quoting Robert Frost again, "That has made all the difference."[3]

FRIENDING

Of all the lessons I'm learning from Parkinson's, what friendship means and requires is certainly one of the more significant ones.

I am not proud of this, but for much of my pre-Parkinson's life I wasn't great with friendships. Don't get me wrong, I had friends; lots of them, in fact. I am grateful for that. Still, I never had the kinds of friendships I have now; and I do not mean only the friendships I enjoy with fellow Parkinson's journeyers. Many of my longtime friendships have also deepened since the beast tapped me on my shoulder.

What I'm talking about are friendships built on trust and risk; loyalty and commitment; generosity and sacrifice; on sharing both joy and sorrow, success and failure, confidence and fear—honestly, consistently, reciprocally.

For nearly three decades, I watched with admiration as Tracey had these kinds of friendships, whether with people she recently met or those that go back to first grade. I saw how life-giving these friendships were for her; how they interweaved with other elements in the fabric of her life. Now, because of Parkinson's, I have these friendships, too. They are one of the gifts that having a progressive, incurable, debilitating, neurologic disease has provided.

Emerson said that, "It is one of the blessings of old friends that you can afford to be stupid with them."[4]

This is true.

But what Tennessee Williams is remembered to have said is also spot on, whether you have Parkinson's, or not.

"Life is partly what we make it, and partly what it is made by the friends we choose."

---

3. Frost, "The Road Not Taken," 119.
4. Emerson, *Journals*, 195.

44

SEASONS OF MY
YOUNG-ONSET PARKINSON'S

SUMMER

As we pull up to the curb and park on a hot summer day in 2003, it catches my eye before anything else. Its tall, thick trunk holds a sprawling canopy reaching halfway across the front yard. Rare in central Austin, this red cedar is why we bought the house. It has had a front row view of significant events in our lives.

Like when I received a Parkinson's diagnosis thirteen years later.

FALL

Exiting the St. David's Hospital parking garage, I begin the one-mile drive home from Dr. T's office. Tracey is outside, tending to one of her beloved flower beds when I pull up in front of our house. She sees me, stands up, and removes her yellow cloth gardening gloves. Dropping them on the ground, she walks to meet me near the sidewalk. Our two Chihuahua mixes, Sunny and Fiona, follow her.

"What did he say?" she asks.

My red eyes moisten. My lips quiver.

"Allan, what did he say?"

"He thinks I have Parkinson's disease."

She covers her mouth with her cupped hands, one on top of the other. She shakes her head as her eyes fill, too.

"Oh, honey . . . No. I can't believe it . . . Is he sure?"

"He said he's pretty sure."

We stand in a silent hug under the canopy of that strong red cedar, which now holds a rope our daughters swing from, the grass under it worn away to hard-packed dirt. I hear a bird chirping quickly and see a young woman pushing a baby in a stroller, but she does not look our way. A gentle breeze blows against our wet faces. It hints at the coming cool of a late central Texas fall.

Our embrace relaxes as Tracey raises her head from my chest and looks at me with her inviting brown eyes. They captured me over a quarter of a century earlier, in a chance meeting in Boston. She wipes her cheeks. Every bit of her 5' 2" slim frame straightens. Her tenacity pops out.

She reaches out for my hands. "I'm actually relieved," she says. "Honestly, when I saw you pulling up, I was worried you had worse news to tell me."

I nod, slowly, and think, "Isn't Parkinson's bad enough?"

"What do you mean?"

"I was worried it might be something horrible," she says. I wasn't going to let myself go to that dark place, but it stayed in the back of my mind . . . and what I mean is that Parkinson's is something we can deal with. It will be OK."

Silence.

"I know. We will get through it. What other choice do we have?"

The branches of that red cedar move, as if to nod along with me.

I force a smile.

She lets go of one hand and we begin walking slowly toward the front door. I tell her about the scan Dr. T is ordering, which will be a couple of weeks away. It's a formality. My body does not feel right and it hasn't for a long time. The reasons are beginning to make sense.

We walk into our safe place, surrounded by photos of those we love most, and sit down together on our green sofa. Tracey folds her body into mine and places her head on my chest.

We sit in silence.

It will be several hours before our girls get home from school.

Looking at pictures of them—on the wall, above the fireplace, atop a row of bookshelves—wondering where I go from here, my eyes turn to our front bay window and I begin to stare at the tree.

WINTER

For nearly ten months, I live locked away in isolation, emotionally if not physically, closely guarding my Parkinson's secret. It weighs on me; eats at me. I need support but fear asking for it.

Then, I have that dream, the one with the strong tree and the wildflowers displaying resilience and radiating beauty, regardless of the wind's strength or direction.

Shortly thereafter, I disclose my illness; first to my parents, then to my children, and then to my boss, friends, and colleagues. I begin trying to use my Parkinson's for good, arm in arm with others seeking to do the same.

SPRING

Three and a half years later, Tracey and I stop on the sidewalk in front of our house. We have just taken Sunny, Fiona, and our newest dog, Hank, for a walk. Still locked down by COVID-19, we talk about the next marathon we hope to run together, which is nearly eight months away. The purple rope hanging from the red cedar catches my eye. A gentle breeze moves it ever so slightly. Beneath it, lush green St. Augustine grass, where hard-packed dirt used to be, reaches toward the sky.

I remember the line from a Shelley poem, "If winter comes, can spring be far behind?"[1]

---

1. Shelley, "Ode to the West Wind."

45

IMPERFECT PEOPLE

"The privilege of a lifetime is to become who you truly are."

—C. G. JUNG

RED FACES

Reaching down below her chair, she attempts discreetly to quiet her two dogs but their playful barks show they could not care less. I see her face reddening as she apologizes profusely.

Twelve of us are on a Zoom call discussing a Phase III clinical trial for a new Parkinson's drug. The dog owner's boss at a large pharmaceutical company has asked her to walk us through the trial's protocol. In all, two patients, a physician, and eight Big Pharma colleagues watch as her discomfort continues for a couple of minutes, which I sense feels to her like hours. When she finishes commenting, she apologizes once more.

"It's not a Zoom meeting until someone's dog barks," I say.

She laughs awkwardly and shakes her head, and then quickly mutes her microphone, pauses her camera, and presumably relocates the dynamic canine duo. After about a minute, she pops back on screen, her face less flush, just in time for her boss to call on her again.

Awkward Zoom moments have become routine. A dog barks, or a cat walks across a computer keyboard, or a child or other family member pops up in the background unaware—in underwear! Unwashed breakfast dishes or piles of clean unfolded laundry sit just within camera shot. Someone's "unmuted" status allows others to hear his daughters arguing over an article of clothing to which they both lay claim.

The Zoom life, which is really the COVID-19 life, humors us and, occasionally, humbles us.

In other words, it *humanizes* us.

DISGUISED FACES

Albert Camus said, "But above all, in order to be, never try to seem."[1] He recognized the strong pull toward maintaining appearances, the power of vanity's grip. Camus observed the masks we wear to hide our true selves from public view, and a propensity to live with red faces over the awkward situations we create, the foibles we reveal, or the imperfections we perceive in ourselves.

Think about how much time and energy we give to presenting the least flawed version of ourselves possible. Consider the work it takes to seem permanently polished, put together, and unblemished, whether in social media posts, automatic "I'm great" responses when asked how we are doing, or in frantic efforts to smooth out the awkwardness tied to barking dogs. The ease with which we default to these glossy self-presentations makes it feel almost natural.

Almost.

But what do we lose along the way?

FACING CHOICES

If having Parkinson's does anything, it confronts you with a realization and a choice. You realize quickly that Parkinson's pushes to the fore your imperfections and awkwardness, right there, in front of God and everybody. Hands shake, feet shuffle, postures stoop, faces mask, voices quiet, speech slurs, and gaits wobble; and that's before you get to what can happen

---

1. Camus, *Notebooks 1935–1951*.

internally: anxiety, depression, constipation, incontinence, insomnia—you get the idea.

Your *choice* is whether a preoccupation with these imperfections and this awkwardness will haunt you, isolate you, and dampen your zest for life, or whether you will recognize that you are really no different from anyone else—flawed, imperfect, human—and then get on with your life.

With time, all of us come face to face with our imperfections, whether we have Parkinson's or not. Bodies begin to sag, droop, or bulge; skin wrinkles; hair grays, falls out, or grows in places you do not want it to; hearing and seeing get more challenging; other unwelcome changes come, too. If we accept these imperfections, these less-than-ideal qualities of life, we can live more authentically, true, and free.

We can also live as happier, more grateful, and more contented people.

Michael J. Fox recognized a certain type of freedom that comes with letting go of vanity, saying, "Now I feel and I say all the time that vanity is, like, long gone. I'm really free of worrying about what I look like, because it's out of my shaky hands. I don't control it. So why would I waste one second of my life worrying about it?"[2]

What if we all adopted this way of thinking about what we can't control, and especially as it relates to our perceived flaws, whether we live with Parkinson's or not? Imagine what it would be like if we could let go of "trying to seem" in order simply "to be."

I can attest to the fact that, with Parkinson's, you discover that the more you try to hide or camouflage your symptoms, the more you try to look put together and unblemished, the more pronounced many of those symptoms become. Maybe this is true for others, too.

Come to think of it, hiding our imperfections is sort of like trying to get two energetic, happy, and playful dogs to stop barking while speaking to a group of imperfect people on Zoom.

2 Fox, "10 Questions."

46

A TEACHER

A TEACHER

It has been about five months since my diagnosis in the fall of 2016, and hardly anyone knows. I'm still preoccupied with living into an uncertain future as a forty-eight-year-old man with young-onset Parkinson's disease, still living in the chronic illness closet walled off by fear and anxiety, sadness and despair.

It's a Sunday afternoon when Norton calls me at home. We are colleagues in the Steve Hicks School of Social Work at The University of Texas at Austin, and he is teaching a course titled "Loss and Grief." Undergoing treatment for cancer, an illness he'd experienced a couple of times before, he had not felt well for weeks, since the semester began, in fact; and he was finding it more difficult to walk and to maintain his energy for a weekly three-hour course.

Before the semester began, I told Norton that I would be ready to assist him if he ever needed the support, and I meant it. I had taught a similar course in previous semesters and was willing to step in at any point. My hope was that the offer would help ease his anxiety about any need to miss class.

No faculty colleague was more conscientious than Norton.

His phone call comes as no surprise. A few days earlier, I saw his wife, Marilyn, who is also a professor in the School of Social Work, and speaking about Norton's decline, she expressed concern about his ability to continue the teaching pace.

Norton tells me that he does not think he can teach on Tuesday and asks if I can cover the class. "I'm planning to be back the following week," he says. "You're not finished with me yet."

I tell him I am happy to fill in for him on Tuesday, and to fill in for him as long as he needs me. We spend a few more minutes going through what he has planned to cover in class that day.

I meet with his class that Tuesday and for the next couple of weeks. Because his health continues to decline, Norton and I then meet at his home and discuss a plan for me to serve as the course instructor for the rest of the semester. We speak at length about his approach to the course and about what he wants students to learn, which I want to honor. At one point in our conversation, he pauses, clears his throat, and says, "I wish I could tell them goodbye."

I think for a moment, and then suggest that we video conference him in to class the next time it meets, so that he can say goodbye and his students can say goodbye to him.

"I'd like that," he says.

LEARNERS

A few days later, we gather for class. The students and I talk about the plan for the day and then have a few minutes before the video conference with Norton begins.

The room becomes silent. Being in their late teens and early twenties, few of these students have come face to face with any person in hospice care, let alone with a teacher in that situation. No one makes eye contact with me as I scan the room.

Then, Norton's face appears on the large screen at the front of the classroom.

He begins leading his class one last time.

With his beloved wife by his side, Norton lies at home in a hospice bed, his head propped up by pillows. Despite his soft scratchy voice, he speaks with deft strength and elegance. As his reassuring tone and winsome spirit take hold, his students relax and listen intently. Several have tears spilling over their young cheekbones.

He greets us and speaks of his sadness over not being able to complete the semester, and of how important teaching in the School of Social Work has been to him. He also notes the irony of his course being on loss and grief, adding, as he chuckles, that he is still trying to figure out who to be mad at about that.

Then he uses his own experience of knowing that the end of his life is drawing nearer to make multiple connections with what he and the students have read, discussed, and wrote about the previous seven or eight weeks.

He teaches us about loss and grief.

LESSONS

I learn other lessons from him, too.

Each of us has purpose for as long as we live. Norton discovered social work education later in life, after a career practicing law; and he remained curious and open to new ideas and experiences. By his own account, he never stopped learning or growing.

We say as much about ourselves and about our take on life with our attitudes and personal commitments as we say with our mouths. Even as his health declined and his energy waned Norton cared about human suffering, his students, and his commitment to equipping them for work that helps people heal.

We are most human when we are most authentic and vulnerable. Speaking to his students from a hospice bed required a level of courage, self-acceptance, and inner strength that continues to inspire me. What a gift he gave those of us there that day. What an example he provided for us to emulate as we live out our own callings, take our own risks, and share our own gifts with others.

When Norton finishes, we have the opportunity to speak to him, each in our own way.

All of us express gratitude, for him and for his teaching. The students voice appreciation for the time they shared. I acknowledge his important contributions to the life and mission of our school, as well as to the social work profession. We reminisce for a brief moment more.

As our time together ends, his students wave to him, with tears again running down their faces. He slowly lifts his arm to wave back as he smiles.

"Take care of yourselves, and thank you," he says.

Wiping my own eyes, I, like Norton, want to be mad at someone. But this anger fades as my gratitude takes a firmer hold.

Because even though death looms, life keeps pushing it away.

47

HEALING BEFORE CURING

June 20, 2020
Dear Will,

I enjoyed meeting you recently, though I wish it were for reasons other than we share a diagnosis of young-onset Parkinson's disease.

You mentioned that you are struggling with how best to cope with your illness, especially in light of being a single father of three young children. I can empathize with your burdens.

Every now and then, it hits me, too. *I have an illness for which there is no cure.* This thought no longer consumes me. Not now. For the first year or so after my diagnosis, though, it did. I thought about Parkinson's almost constantly—day and night. I even had dreams about it.

It is better now, but Parkinson's still never leaves my awareness. My body reminds me of its slowly tightening grip every time I move. Even though the medicine works like a charm, and I am grateful it does, I never feel Parkinson's-free. I know you can relate to this experience.

So every now and then, it hits me: *Progressive. Degenerative. Incurable. Parkinson's.*

Evidently, a similar realization hits you. Given that you received the diagnosis less than a year ago, I understand you being, as you said, full of questions.

When we met, you asked me one of those questions to which I have given more thought. *How do you deal with knowing you are going to have this disease for the rest of your life?*

I think I understand where the question comes from. In fact, I asked it myself when Parkinson's took up residence in my brain.

Actually, Will, I believe that eventually we will have a cure for Parkinson's; and I would not bet against it happening in our lifetime. As you may know, we are close, very close, to significant breakthroughs. Smart people I trust—doctors, researchers, persons with Parkinson's (PwP) alike—tell me this; and they are straight talkers.[1] Therefore, I help raise money for a cure. I try to educate people who can help with efforts to find a cure. Around the world, 10 million people clamor for a cure and I am one of them.

Let me be clear. By *cure*, I mean medications or other interventions that allow us to live symptom-free, which is not the same thing as eradicating the disease process. Oh, I hope for this, too; believe me. But I'll settle for living symptom-free for the rest of my life.

At the same time, I cannot base my happiness, or my inner peace, on there being a cure for Parkinson's. Basing my happiness on finding a cure would mean wasting my one and only life, and blowing opportunities to experience joy, meaning, and purpose each day with those I love. Looking over the horizon inevitably takes my eyes away from beautiful, sacred, and life-giving experiences and humans that dwell right in front of me.

What is the alternative?

For me, it helps to balance the energy I give to finding a *cure* with energy I give to finding ways to *heal*. By healing, I mean restoring and preserving a sense of wholeness and personal integrity, even as the Parkinson's beast indwells.[2] You can heal without having a cure. I have learned this from Parkinson's.

For me, healing begins with hope, with believing that Parkinson's has invited me to make a persistent, stubborn commitment to being hopeful. Each day, I pledge my hopefulness, saying to myself, sometimes aloud,

> *I am grateful for another day.*
> *I will do my best to make it good.*
> *I will focus on my strengths.*
> *I will be hopeful.*

1. PwP is an abbreviation for person with Parkinson's.

2. This definition of healing comes from philosopher S. Kay Toombs, who lives with her own chronic, progressive illness—multiple sclerosis.

My choice to begin each day this way follows from a belief that hope helps me savor life in the moment, *today*, and to recognize that today is all any of us have.

I hold fast to other sources of hope, too: family and friends; what I have, not what I lack; what I can still do, not only in spite of Parkinson's, but *because* of it; and what brings me the greatest sense of *purpose*—teaching, writing, and leading in a school of social work; and, of course, being a father.

I want to thank you, Will. Your question helped me realize something I had not been as keenly aware of. Making sense out of having Parkinson's, and being confident that my having it matters, regardless of how it turns out, regardless of whether we find a cure, helps me find joy in the present. This joy feeds back into my hope.

William Butler Yeats said, "Things reveal themselves passing away."[3] Living with Parkinson's disease feels as if things are passing away, slowly but surely. Movement slows, muscles tighten, cramp, and sometimes spasm and hurt, fingers and hands become less steady, balance wanes, sleep fades, other changes come.

I suspect you know this, Will.

Still, there is hope.

While some things pass away with Parkinson's, it reveals other extraordinary things that matter.

Herein lies the healing.

Sincerely,
Allan

3. Yeats, *Collected Works,* 297.

48

A LETTER TO MY DAUGHTER ON
RESILIENCE

———————

May 25, 2020
Dear Meredith,

Earlier this evening, as you worked on your middle school graduation speech, I listened and watched with a full heart.

After rehearsing an idea, you would pause, look up toward the ceiling, and then, peering back at the screen, tap quickly on your laptop's keys. The tip of your tongue protruded slightly between your lips as you picked up the pace. That's always been your "tell," how I know you are deep in thought.

It took me back to when you were about five years old. That's when we started our practice of talking about meaningful things as I sat at the foot of your bed. Then and now, you are wiser than your years.

Now fourteen, you are about give the commencement speech. Wow! What an honor.

And what a difference a year makes.

Last year at this time, in a different school, you ran into a buzz saw of adolescent betrayal. And you chose not to dwell on others' actions but to focus on who you want to be.

You often joke about my liking philosophy and quoting philosophers, so here I go.

A nineteenth-century German philosopher named Friedrich Nietzsche once wrote, "What doesn't kill me makes me stronger."[1] This might not always be true; after all, it can be hard to see how strength could follow from the most severe hardships we face.

On the other hand, I think Nietzsche was right to recognize that people have the ability to build something called *resilience*, to bounce back from a difficult experience or crisis and to be as strong, or stronger, than ever before—to be resilient.

We talk a lot about resilience in social work, and even teach classes at Texas on how to help people build more of it for themselves as they grow. It is a good thing to have, no doubt.

As you read your speech to me, I realized that you were talking about this kind of growth, about resilience. You spoke about opportunities for growth shared by all of the eighth graders graduating and heading to high school, and opportunities for any of us, really, who need to bounce back from painful or disorienting experiences.

This is what you said.

"It is so important to continue to be kind, compassionate, and welcoming to others no matter where you are. The world needs more peacemakers, advocates, creators, and thinkers. So wherever you go, I hope you will bring the values apparent here [at this school] with you; values such as kindness, compassion, advocacy, creativity, curiosity, a passion for learning, and a commitment to making the world a better place. Please treat others the way you want to be treated. As high school students, we will continue the journey of deciding what type of people we want to be, and what contributions we want to make to the world. I truly hope that among your many contributions, integrity, respect, justice, and equity will be prevalent."

You concluded with these words: "Take a moment and think [about] where you're going. Wherever your path takes you, I urge you to remember the values that are so prevalent here. Remember, as Mahatma Gandhi said, 'You must be the change you want to see in the world.'"

I want to say thank you, my love. What you shared about your hard experience last year, and how you talked about it motivating you this year, well, it taught me some things about living and growing, including with Parkinson's.

- Life does not always go as planned.

1. Nietzsche, *Twilight of the Idols*, 6.

- Disappointments and heartaches can paralyze us or motivate us.

- Growth can follow setbacks.

- When facing adversity, we do well to focus on our strengths.

- The world needs more peacemakers, advocates, creators, and thinkers.

- Integrity, respect, justice, and equity are timeless and essential values, no matter our age.

- We have to be the change we want to see in the world.

- We are never too young, or too old, to be this change.

- You can learn a lot from a kid.

Your reflections also reminded me of something Michael J. Fox has said, "One's dignity may be assaulted, vandalized and cruelly mocked, but it can never be taken away unless it is surrendered."[2]

I'm proud of you.

Love,
Dad
P.S. Remind me to tell you about Aristotle.

2. See Berhnhard, *How to Live Well,* 271.

49

STEPPING UP TO THE PLATE

Who knew that my first childhood love, playing baseball, would help me live with Parkinson's disease?

1980

Ken and I are teammates on our sixth-grade baseball team and he is awful at baseball. Tall and skinny, he lacks muscular coordination. Walking on his tiptoes, he bounces along with the agility of a young colt learning to walk. Sometimes, like a colt, he appears on the verge of falling flat on his face.

Ken is friendly but also shy, and he never wants attention. Everyone on the team likes him and appreciates his steadfast efforts to improve and to contribute. In fact, he motivates the rest of us to work harder ourselves. In this way, he is an unlikely leader.

Despite his efforts, Ken gets little playing time. If not for the league's requirement that coaches play each kid at least two innings in every game, he would hardly ever get on the field. Batting presents the biggest challenge. He *always* strikes out. Always! Usually without making contact with any ball thrown to him. More times than not, a ball pitched to him reaches the catcher's mitt before Ken swings his bat.

STRIKING OUT

A predictable feeling of dread grabs me when I see Ken trot onto the field. I think my teammates and all of our parents feel this same dread. Ken must feel it, too. Practice after practice, game after game.

We say things like, "Keep your head up," "You'll get 'em next time," and "Good effort, Ken." We all want so badly for him to succeed.

Ken's frustration level wears on him; you can see it. More and more, he slams his bat to the ground when he strikes out, turning its end into the dirt like a corkscrew. Sometimes he kicks the dirt as he walks back to the dugout, his head held low and shaking firmly back and forth as if to say, "No. No. No."

It's our next-to-the-last game, and after striking out again and verbally bashing himself as he walks back to the dugout, Ken can no longer hold back his tears. Laying his bat down, he walks briskly to the far end of the bench, places his sweaty face in his dirty, slender, boyish hands, and weeps. Trying desperately not to cry, his body shakes noticeably.

All of us try not to stare, not knowing what else to do.

After a couple of minutes, Ken lifts his head, gives his now dirt-streaked face a long wipe with his forearm and the back of his hand, and trots out to his place in right field, where he completes the inning and finishes the game.

THE LAST AT BAT

It's now the following Saturday, the last game of the season, and Ken is inserted dutifully into the line-up in the eighth inning. With it being our team's turn to bat, he is second in the order. Our teammate Corey just got on base with a walk.

Ken approaches the batter's box. That familiar feeling of dread grabs me as my thoughts return to the previous game.

On the very first pitch, Ken swings the bat and misses. The catcher's leather mitt pops. The same thing happens with the second pitch. Two strikes.

On the third pitch, Ken swings the bat and makes contact with the ball, which bloops over the second baseman's head and into right field!

With eyes a large as saucers, Ken takes off running toward first base on his tiptoes, his long arms pumping back and forth while his gangly body works to stay upright. He reaches first base and *finally* gets a hit.

The expression on his face tells the story, one that remains embossed in my memory. Several of us take a quick couple of steps out of the dugout, ready to swarm the field in celebration, before our coach stops us.

When two other teammates both get a hit and Ken crosses home plate to score, the entire team encircles him and we shout, "Ken! Ken! Ken! Ken!" He holds his arms high in the air and his head almost as high. We all have our arms around each other. A pervasive joy hovers over the red Georgia dirt for several minutes, and no one wants it to end.

I have a palpable sense of what I can only call divine compassion; and I am grateful.

2020

Forty years and a Parkinson's diagnosis later, my eyes still moisten when I think about Ken—about his struggle, his strength, his hit at the end of the season. I can still see him wipe away his tears, straighten his back, and exhale as, once again, he steps up to the plate, tightens his grip, and invites me to follow his lead.

50

ONE THING

CLIFF

"There should be a rule that you only get one thing!" My friend Cliff makes this statement as we visit by Zoom. Late in the evening, he has hat head and three- or four-day gray stubble. His lament comes from a vulnerable place—one of anxiety and fear, existential angst, and both physical and emotional fatigue.

His Parkinson's symptoms with a COVID-19 overlay are significant.

Cliff learned a few days earlier of his positive COVID test results, and as he strains almost incessantly to discern how he became infected—"I was so careful"—and with whom he might have come into contact—"I hope I didn't give it to anyone"—an insidious virus gripping much of the world is in a standoff with his body.

New to club PD, Cliff received a Parkinson's diagnosis just a couple of months ago. As many of us do, he bobs up and down in a rough sea of symptoms, working as hard as he can to figure out how to calm them, how to live with them: hour by hour, day by day. Now, he has COVID-19, too—an unexpected gale force storm to ride out.

"I know," I say. "Parkinson's alone is all-consuming."

MITCH AND CURLY

Later that night, as I thought more about our conversation, and especially of Cliff's comment—*There should be a rule that you only get one thing*—I remembered a scene in a 1991 movie titled *City Slickers*. It starred Billy Crystal, who plays Mitch Robbins, and Jack Palance, a rugged, seasoned cowboy named Curly. Fending off threats of a midlife crisis, Mitch and his two friends, all of them urbanites, embark on a two-week cattle drive from New Mexico to Colorado, where they meet Curly. On a break from lassoing errant cattle, he confronts Mitch with an existential question.

"Do you know what the secret of life is?" Curly asks.

Silence.

Holding up one finger, Curly says, "This. One thing. Just one thing. You stick to that and the rest don't mean shit."

"But what's the 'one thing'?" asks Mitch.

Smiling, Curly says, "That's what you have to figure out."

US

Like Curly, Parkinson's has an uncanny ability to lasso and pull you into a new reflective space, and there it beckons you to figure out things. Many questions linger and lure you toward hoping, if not believing, that all you have to do is discover that *one thing*—that which, when figured out, offers up, once and for all, the answer to the questions that take up residence in both your conscious and unconscious mind from the moment you get the diagnosis. Live questions. Pressing questions. Questions having to do with *one thing*—namely, how do I live with this illness?

Of course, many questions live within this larger question. Questions of meaning, values, and purpose; of priorities, passions, and hope. Medical questions, relationship questions, insurance questions, financial questions, parenting questions . . . the list goes on.

So fundamentally human, our answers, even if provisional, point to something we must need in order to keep weathering Parkinson's storms, and to keep searching, if not for the secret of life, then for something that can help us with the key to living well, and meaningfully, and with joy.

Evidently, what Parkinson's, COVID-19, and midlife crises share, at least in my free-associating brain, is that they put before us enduring questions, many of which relate to personal values, priorities, passions, and goals—to what we most want and need.

Which gets us back to what we have to figure out, our *one thing*—how we live with this illness, and how we can stick to our tenacious commitment to rise each day empowered by this *one thing*, so that the rest of PD don't mean shit.

51

AESOP AND MOSES

GOING TO SCHOOL

In the winter of 1996, I sit with three other students in a windowless office on the first floor of New York Hospital-Cornell Medical Center, located on New York's Upper East Side. All of us will graduate in a few months from Columbia University's School of Social Work.

We have gathered this late morning with our supervisor, Dr. Sonia Austrian, as we do each week, to discuss our work with clients in the Employee Assistance Program that she oversees.

As social work interns providing employees with short-term counseling, we benefit from hearing each other's perspectives on how best to support those who, in varying degrees, struggle with *something*. Those struggles include depression and anxiety, as well as concerns about relationships, parenting, illness, finances, and other experiences we call problems in living. We interns meet weekly to debrief and to receive feedback as we learn what to do and not to do as budding counselors.

Discussing one particular case involving a young man with relationship difficulties, my classmates exchange perspectives on his experience, problems, and needs.

"He clearly needs longer-term therapy," Steven argues. "We are just scratching the surface after meeting four times."

"I agree," says Jodi. "He is really struggling."

I listen for several minutes to their back-and-forth assessments and proposed treatment plans. Sonia keeps looking at me, waiting, I assume, for my response. Finally, her large blue eyes open wider than usual as she looks my way.

Clearing my throat, I say, "It occurs to me that it could be a lot worse."

Jodi and Steven look stunned. Sonia laughs. "Leave it to Allan to find a positive take on all of this," she says.

ASSESSING IDEAS

I am not sure whether her tone was affirming or critical. Either way, my response revealed an approach to dealing with hardships, an approach to life, really, that had been instilled in me and which I embraced.

I suppose I still do.

Which raises the question of whether it is helpful or hurtful to think in these terms—to follow Aesop and take an "It-can-alway-be-worse" attitude toward human struggles, whether our own or others'.

This perspective risks being hurtful when it prompts us to minimize, gloss over, or worse, dismiss human pain. In this case, "It can always be worse" can mean, "I don't notice or affirm your struggles, suffering, and need of support."

On the other hand, this take on adversity has benefits. The view that, in many cases, the magnitude of our difficulties, while significant, distressing, and surely deserving of care and support, nevertheless may not be as catastrophic as we might otherwise assume—this view can help us cope and actually feel better.

Here's how this perspective often plays out for me.

On days when I am more symptomatic or I feel less well, it helps me to remember what I have that is positive and good in my life *and* what prevents me from struggling more severely than I do. Things like, I have a steady job and access to excellent medical care, medication, and insurance that pays for both. That I can rely on a loving partner, my kind and compassionate children and parents, a supportive boss and colleagues, generous friends and neighbors. And that I have many sisters and brothers in the Parkinson's community, too, who willingly offer their encouragement and share their own ways of coping with PD's effects. On my difficult days, I am still quite fortunate to have all of this, and more, which, incidentally, I know many others do not have. Far from dismissing my struggles, remembering the good fortune I enjoy actually serves to help me feel better and to maintain a positive outlook on life with Parkinson's.

LEARNING A CRAFT

Living with illness can become a craft of sorts, meaning we can get better at it the more practice we have. We learn tricks of the trade that help improve us as craftspeople. For me, getting better at the craft includes balancing the desire and need to have my struggles recognized and validated, on the one hand, and to keep them in proper perspective, on the other. This proper perspective includes reminding myself that not only could things be worse for me, but that things are already worse for others.

I don't know if this perspective works for you, but it just might help if you give it a try.

If I could go back to that moment during my internship with Jodi, Steven, and Sonia, I would tell them I like the way Kirk Douglass put it: "No matter how bad things are, they can always be worse. So what if my stroke left me with a speech impediment? Moses had one, and he did all right."[1]

1. Sager, "Kirk Douglas."

52

FRIENDSHIPS, OLD AND NEW

"Piglet sidled up to Pooh from behind.
"Pooh!" he whispered.
"Yes, Piglet?"
"Nothing," said Piglet, taking Pooh's paw. "I just wanted to be sure of you."

—A.A. MILNE

OLD FRIENDS

It's 1980, near the end of my sixth-grade year, and my parents and I are leaving Plano, Texas, a budding suburb of Dallas where new housing developments spring up like popcorn in the flat north Texas landscape.

A brisk, cool March breeze blows, making the flagpole outside Haggard Middle School clang.

I see my dad's car parked at the curb, pointed toward Atlanta. He and my mom sit patiently in the front seat, allowing me the time I need to say my goodbyes after the day's final school bell rings. In a few days, I will start at my new school.

I see Ryan and Tony, and we part quickly in the way twelve-year-old boys do—saying something like, "Stay cool, man" before they ride off on their BMX bikes doing wheelies down the street. Then, I see Craig and

Clay, my next-door neighbor Staci, and a few others whose names I cannot recall. They wish me well and pledge to stay in touch, but this is difficult in the days before email and the Internet.

Looking down the rows of bike racks, my eyes flit to the heavy sea of adolescent kids that now surrounds the school. I scan it for Tracy, my close friend since fourth grade. We often sit next to each other in class, get in trouble for talking at the wrong times, pass notes, and share homework answers. For her tenth birthday, I rode my bike to Zee's Tees and picked out a light blue hoodie and had a sparkling rainbow-colored decal ironed onto it. It is the first time I remember saving my money to buy a gift for a friend. She wore the hoodie all the time.

Smart, interesting, and funny, Tracy is among the first people I recall feeling sure of as a friend.

Now forty years later, I think of all of this, and more, as I log on to Zoom before speaking with her.

NEW FRIENDS

Earlier that same day, I had a Zoom call with Ethan, one of my newer closest friends. He and I have Parkinson's disease, and we met a couple of years ago through the Michael J. Fox Foundation for Parkinson's Research. When we get together, we talk about Parkinson's, of course, and how we're each doing—with meds, movement, sleep, and other challenges—but we also talk about running a next marathon together, politics, work, and our families—the kinds of things friends talk about because they're meaningful and personal.

What Tracy and Ethan have in common are ties that bind; ties of friendship characterized by risk and trust, authenticity and openness, freedom and laughter; the ties that unite human beings in ways that enliven their souls and offer assurances that endure. These ties often begin in childhood, but they can form at any age. In fact, I count the friendships I have made with others on the Parkinson's path—with people like Ethan—as one of the unexpected gifts this illness has offered me.

Henri Nouwen understood friendship more keenly than most. He writes, "When we honestly ask ourselves which persons in our lives mean the most to us, we often find that it is those who, instead of giving advice, solutions, or cures, have chosen rather to share our pain and touch our wounds with a warm and tender hand. The friend who can be silent with us in a moment of despair or confusion, who can stay with us in an hour of grief and bereavement, who can tolerate not knowing, not curing, not healing and face with us the reality of our powerlessness, that is a friend who cares."[1]

SURE FRIENDS

I think I have gotten better at friendship since Parkinson's took up residence in my brain. I have become more like I was in my childhood. Eager to share another's struggles and willing to share my own. Comfortable in the difficulty of silence, ambiguity, and, yes, in some instances, my powerlessness. We have so much less control than we assume that we do. Parkinson's teaches us this. In fact, thanks to Parkinson's, like Milne's Piglet, I am less enamored with control, and more comfortable with, and comforted by, merely reaching out to my friends for assurance, and with them reaching out to me.

Which reminds me, again, of Tracy.

In the fifth grade, at Tony's house, my hand and arm accidentally went through a glass pane in a French door, which required many stitches and my missing a few days of school. Tracy made a card for me that said, "I'm sorry you cut your arm" and urged me to "Get back to school!" She rode her bike to my house with another friend and gave the card to me with some candy. The kind of thing a friend does, whether old or new.

My arm healed and I got back to school. The following year, I would make that drive with my parents to Atlanta and Tracy would move to Houston with her family. Many years passed before we reconnected, but it felt like we just picked up where we left off.

Even though he was not there, I have a feeling Ethan will understand. In fact, I'm sure of it.

1. Nouwen, *Out of Solitude*, 38.

53

A HOPEFUL FUTURE

FUTURE DOCS

The fifty or so youthful faces begin to appear on my laptop's screen just before 8 AM, all of them belonging to first-year medical students. Their instructor and my University of Texas colleague, a neurologist, has spent several weeks introducing these students to basic neurology and neurologic illnesses. Having invited me to speak with them just prior to their final exam, to share my story of living with Parkinson's, he has noted that I will be the first "real patient" they have met in the context of their medical education.

No pressure there.

Seeing several of them take sips of coffee or Diet Coke to help prop open sleepy eyes, I begin recapping my story.

It started with a slight tremor in my left index finger, which led to visiting my primary care doctor . . . Next came a misdiagnosis by one neurologist before receiving an accurate diagnosis from another . . . Then came nearly a year of life in the Parkinson's closet, before finally telling my parents, children, and colleagues . . .

Speaking of the newfound freedom that followed, and of my commitment to trying to tame the Parkinson's beast and use it for good, I then offer a few words of wisdom to these budding MDs. Some of that wisdom comes from friends, whose input I had solicited prior to meeting with the class.

"If I'm your patient, focus not only on the dopamine levels in my brain, but also on whether I will dance with my daughters at their weddings. Focus not merely on my symptoms, but on my passions and contributions. See me as someone living with Parkinson's and not as a person defined by it."

Several of the students nod their heads, and so does my colleague as I continue.

"You are an exceptionally gifted group of people that will have opportunities to make a difference in people's lives that not many of us ever have. So, do not leave here knowing merely how to treat disease. Leave here knowing how to treat human beings with stories to tell and with new chapters left to write. Only then will you have an exemplary medical education."

PRESENTLY HOPEFUL

A few days later, having reflected on our time together, I realized I was speaking to those students about hope. People with illnesses such as Parkinson's want and need to have hope; and our physicians have the opportunity to participate in our search, even to be a conduit for it, as they humanize their care.

Wendell Berry puts it this way in "A Poem of Hope":

> It is hard to have hope. It is harder as you grow old,
> for hope must not depend on feeling good
> and there is the dream of loneliness at absolute midnight.
> You also have withdrawn belief in the present reality
> of the future, which surely will surprise us,
> and hope is harder when it cannot come by prediction
> any more than by wishing. But stop dithering.
> The young ask the old to hope. What will you tell them?
> Tell them at least what you say to yourself.[1]

I tell myself I am a hopeful person by nature, and this is true. But I think I aspire to the virtue of hope as much as I embody it or live tethered to its power. I am hopeful in the way that Kierkegaard conceived of it, namely, I can see possibilities and envision a future.[2]

1. Berry, "VI," 91. Though untitled, many refer to this poem as "A Poem of Hope."

2. Søren Kierkegaard (1813–1855) was a Danish philosopher who wrote extensively about ethics, religion, and what today would be called psychology. Often identified as a forebearer of existentialism, I learned much about his perspective on hope from my colleague, David J. Gouwens. See his *Kierkegaard as Religious Thinker*, 154–55.

I have always been this way.

On the one hand, as Wendell Berry has taught me, I try hard to live mostly in the present because the future does not exist; the present is what we have. On the other hand, I recognize that, throughout history, persons facing illness, disappointment, loss, violence, poverty, discrimination, and tragedies of many sorts have pointed to the ability to see better possibilities—to *hope*—as the close ally to perseverance and even survival.

To hope in the face of despair prevents us from succumbing to darkness. Living in the present as if you *have* a future, one marked by a meaningful life that *only* you can live, produces energy and resolve in the face of current challenges. Parkinson's disease has prompted my re-examination of hope, not because I have lost a measure of it but because I want to make damn certain I understand it *and* that it has substance and weight.

A HOPEFUL FUTURE

What a difference four years can make. Since my diagnosis in the fall of 2016, I have gone from being heartbroken, blanketed with anxiety, and assuming my life was essentially over at the age of forty-eight, to recognizing that in some ways life has just begun. I have gone from despair to hope. Now, speaking to future doctors about my experiences with Parkinson's and my hopes for the future—for me and 10 million others—well, this makes my heart *sing*.

What was so lovely about this experience with these students is that the present and future collided. I caught myself several times wondering if one of them would, in a few years, discover a new Parkinson's drug, or a new way to use deep brain stimulation, or find some treatment not yet even thought of, such as the Holy Grail of disease-modifying therapies that might stop the beast in its tracks.

I caught myself thinking about an exciting future that will surprise us.

I caught myself experiencing hope.

54

MY FAVORITE DAY

NORMALCY

"When will life be normal again?" My fourteen-year-old daughter Meredith asks this question, her large brown eyes peering over the top of a blue plaid cloth mask. Their half squint, as well as her tone, tell the story.

Meredith, her sister Holly, and I are on our bikes. It's early evening in mid-July, roughly four months into the COVID-19 global pandemic, and the temperatures in central Texas have reached their customary high 90s. Thick air blankets us as we ride slowly through our neighborhood, a nightly antidote to a spreading monotony. The masks stick to our sweaty faces as we pedal through weighty air.

Meredith and Holly have already faced the disruptions of online school and the disappointments of cancelled birthday parties. They have accommodated the need to move most of their adolescent lives into a virtual space—everything from piano lessons and dance class to doctor's appointments and the lion's share of friendships. They long to see their grandparents, to host sleepovers and pool parties, to travel as we typically do on summer vacation, to approximate former lives and their rhythms, which, for us, includes an abundance of privilege.

Listening to Meredith's lament, which I know scores of others share, reminds me of Joan Didion's similar question, "How could this have happened when everything was normal?"[1]

DISRUPTION

In the first months following my Parkinson's diagnosis, I asked similar questions. *When will life be normal again? How could this have happened?* For forty-eight years, I felt well, took no medicine, and made plans for a future I naively imagined already existed, was predictable, and which I took for granted.

When do I get back to that life? When everything was so normal?

As hard as I tried, I could not get away from this answer to Meredith's question: *It is not going to be normal again, if by this we mean exactly as it was before.*

Of course, in some ways, this is an extraordinarily sad and even gloomy conclusion to come to; but it is an honest one informed by the experiences of multiple and profound losses that so many of us continue to sustain in this pandemic. The most severe losses include the ability to work and make a living, permanent injury to the body's systems, and, of course, the death of a friend, family member, or other loved one.

But other losses need recognition, too, such as the loss of feeling human touch and of seeing human faces; the loss of birthday parties, and of shared work spaces, worship spaces, classrooms, and athletic fields; the loss of commencement exercises, bat mitzvahs, weddings, and funerals, among many, many others.

We are losing some of our most fundamental human qualities and experiences, those that not only ground us in normalcy but also tether us to one another in the most basic but necessary ways. Therefore, any new normal has to include the hard work of mourning, of recognizing and accepting our losses, individually and collectively, as a first step toward integrating them into our lives.

Mourning takes time, of course, as well as hard emotional work, and it is difficult to begin this work when we still have no end in sight with respect to the pandemic's toll. We are all still losing to COVID-19, some of us in incomprehensible, not to mention irreplaceable, ways.

---

1. Didion, *The Year of Magical Thinking*, 68.

The same holds true, by the way, for a life with Parkinson's, with any chronic illness, really. Each day, the illness takes from you, from those you love, from a future that in reality does not yet exist but on which you want to hang a lot of hope. It's difficult for anyone to live like we do, incurring so much loss.

A NEW NORMAL

Still, there are some things to hold onto that offer hope. A great gift of living with uncertainty is that it summons you not to take normalcy for granted, and it invites you to recognize the privilege that so often links with questions such as, "How could this have happened when everything was normal?"

Not only this, but when you can no longer count on things being normal again, whether because of illness, a pandemic, or other hardship, you can mourn what has been lost, set new expectations, and recalibrate your heart. Then, you can strive to live expectantly and with gratitude once again—in a new normal.

How do you do this? One way is to mourn what you have lost while also recognizing what you have gained.

In my case, my family takes bike rides through the neighborhood with masks, our own share of losses and questions, fears and anxieties, anger and lament, grief and sorrow. We also roll with unanticipated gifts—of time, intentionality, connection, gratitude, safety, provision—of being alive.

The same can be true for those on the Parkinson's ride.

Which reminds me of when Meredith and Holly were much younger and we read together before bed.

> "What day is it?" asked Pooh.
> "It's today," squeaked Piglet.
> "My favorite day," said Pooh.[2]

2. Cited in Sinclair, *Life Span,* 309.

BIBLIOGRAPHY

Ali, Muhammad. "21 of Muhammad Ali's Best Quotes." *Parade,* February 22, 2014. https://parade.com/264190/viannguryen/50th-anniversary-of-liston-clay-fight-15-of-muhammad-alis-best-quotes/.

Angelou, Maya. *All God's Children Need Traveling Shoes.* New York: Vintage, 1991.

Berhnhard, Toni. *How to Live Well with Chronic Pain and Illness: A Mindful Guide.* Somerville, MA: Wisdom, 2015.

Berry, Wendell. "VI." In *Leavings,* 91. Berkeley, CA: Counterpoint, 2010.

———. *What Are People For?* Berkeley, CA: Counterpoint, 2010.

Brooks, David. "Making Modern Toughness." *New York Times,* August 30, 2016.

Brown, Brené. *Rising Strong.* New York: Random House, 2015.

———. "Shame v. Guilt." *Brené Brown,* January 14, 2013. https://brenebrown.com/blog/2013/01/14/shame-v-guilt/.

Camus, Albert. *Notebooks 1935–1951.* Boston: Da Capo, 1998.

———. *The Plague.* New York: Vintage, 1991.

Carel, Havi. *Illness.* New York: Routledge, 2013.

———. *Phenomenology of Illness.* New York: Oxford University Press, 2016.

"CDC 1 in 4 US adults live with a disability." *Center for Disease Control and Prevention.* https://www.cdc.gov/media/releases/2018/p0816-disability.html.

Cicero. "Pro Plancio." *Britannica.* https://www.britannica.com/topic/Pro-Plancio.

"Conditions that Mimic Parkinson's." *Parkinson's Foundation.* https://www.parkinson.org/Understanding-Parkinsons/Diagnosis/Conditions-that-Mimic-Parkinsons.

Day, Dorothy. *The Long Loneliness.* New York: Harper and Row, 1952.

Didion, Joan. *The Year of Magical Thinking.* New York: Alfred A. Knopf, 2005.

"The Doctor Won't See You Now? Study: US Facing a Neurologist Shortage." *American Academy of Neurology.* https://www.aan.com/PressRoom/Home/PressRelease/1178.

Dostoevsky, Fyodor. *The Brothers Karamazov.* New York: Bantam, 1984.

Dwyer, Jim "Confronting a Stranger, for Art." *The New York Times,* April 4, 2010. https://www.nytimes.com/2010/04/04/nyregion/04about.html.

Emerson, Ralph Waldo. "Friendship." In *The Essays of Ralph Waldo Emerson,* 111–28. Cambridge, MA: Harvard University Press, 1979.

————. *The Journals and Miscellaneous Notebooks of Ralph Waldo Emerson*. Cambridge, MA: President and Fellows of Harvard College, 1982.

————. "Self-Reliance." In *The Collected Works of Ralph Waldo Emerson,* vol. 2, 25–52. Cambridge, MA: Harvard University Press, 1972.

Erikson, Erik H. *Insight and Responsibility*. New York: Norton, 1994.

Foucault, Michel. *The Birth of the Clinic*. New York: Routledge, 1989.

Fox, Michael J. "10 Questions for Michael J. Fox." *Time,* April 27, 2009. http://content. time.com/time/subscriber/article/0,33009,1891739,00.html.

————. "Michael J. Fox at 50: 'I Don't Look at Life as a Battle.'" *Parade,* April 1, 2012. https://parade.com/103452/dotsonrader/01-michael-j-fox/.

Frankel, Viktor E. *Man's Search for Meaning*. Boston: Beacon, 1992.

Frost, Robert. "The Road Not Taken." In *The Poetry of Robert Frost*, rev. ed., 105. New York: Holt, 2002.

————. "A Time to Talk." In *The Poetry of Robert Frost*, rev. ed., 124. New York: Holt, 2002.

"Getting to Equal: The Disability Inclusion Advantage." *Accenture*. https://www.accenture. com/t20181108T081959Z__w__/us-en/_acnmedia/PDF-89/Accenture-Disability-Inclusion-Research-Report.pdf#zoom=50.

Goleman, Daniel. "Erikson, in His Own Old Age, Expands His View of Life." *New York Times,* June 14, 1988. https://archive.nytimes.com/www.nytimes.com/books/99/08/22/ specials/erikson-old.html?scp=161&sq=old%25people&st=Search.

Gouwens, David J. *Kierkegaard as Religious Thinker*. Cambridge: Cambridge University Press, 1996.

Hawking, Stephen W. "The Science of Second-Guessing." *New York Times Magazine,* December 12, 2004. https://www.nytimes.com/2004/12/12/magazine/the-science-of-second-guessing.html.

James, Henry. *The Wings of the Dove*. New York: Charles Scribner's Sons, 1902.

Joplin, Janis. "Me and Bobby McGee." *Pearl*. Columbia Records, 1971.

Josephs, Ray. "Robert Frost's Secret." *This Week Magazine*, September 1954, 1.

Kierkegaard, Søren. *Either/Or*. Part II. Princeton, NJ: Princeton University Press, 1987.

Kinsley, Michael. *Old Age: A Beginner's Guide*. New York: Crown, 2016.

Lamott, Anne. *Plan B: Further Thoughts on Faith*. New York: Riverhead, 2005.

Levinas, Emmanuel. "Signature." No. 294 in *Difficult Freedom: Essays on Judaism,* Baltimore: Johns Hopkins University Press, 1997.

————. *Totality and Infinity*. Pittsburgh: Dusquesne University Press, 1999.

Lewis, C. S. "To Sir Henry Willink." In *Letters of C. S. Lewis*, edited by W. H. Lewis, 483–85. New York: Harcourt, 1966.

McCourt, Frank. *Teacher Man*. New York: Scribner, 2006.

Marina Abramovic Institute. "Marina Abramovic on the Artist Is Present." *Vimeo,* 2010. https://vimeo.com/72711715.

Messer, William, ed. *The Sayings of Epicurus*. Rio de Janeiro: Bibliomundi, 2021.

Mitchell, Margaret. *Gone with the Wind*. New York: Pocket, 1998.

Morrison, Toni. *Song of Solomon*. New York: Vintage, 1977.

Morum, Malka, and Joni Mitchell. *Joni Mitchell: Both Sides Now*. New York: Ominbus, 2001.

Nietzsche, Friedrich. *Twilight of the Idols*. New York: Hackett, 1997.

Nouwen, Henri J. M. *Out of Solitude*. Notre Dame, IN: Ave Maria, 2004.

Parker, Bret. "Parkinson's Disease: The Last Workplace Secret." *Forbes*, May 12, 2012. https://www.forbes.com/sites/randalllane/2012/03/12/the-last-workplace-secret/#7370145b62fe.

"Parkinson's disease: New drugs and treatments, but where are the doctors?" *University of Florida News*. https://news.ufl.edu/articles/2017/09/parkinsons-disease-new-drugs-and-treatments-but-where-are-the-doctors.html.

Pessoa, Fernando. *The Book of Disquiet*. Rhinebeck, NY: Sheep Meadow, 1996.

Plato. *The Republic of Plato*. 3rd ed. Translated by Allan Bloom, Introduction by Adam Kirsch. New York: Basic, 2016.

Robins, Jill, ed. *Is It Righteous to Be? Interviews with Emmanuel Levinas.*, Stanford, CA: Stanford University Press, 2001.

Sacks, Oliver. "My Own Life." *The New York Times*, February 2, 2015. https://www.nytimes.com/2015/02/19/opinion/oliver-sacks-on-learning-he-has-terminal-cancer.html.

Sager, Mike. "Kirk Douglas: What I've Learned." *Esquire*, January 29, 2007. https://www.esquire.com/entertainment/interviews/a1585/learned-kirk-douglas-0401/.

Schrag, A., Y. Ben-Shlomo, N. Quinn. "How Valid is the Clinical Diagnosis of Parkinson's Disease in the Community?" *Journal of Neurology, Neurosurgery & Psychiatry*, vol. 73, 2002. https://jnnp.bmj.com/content/73/5/529.

Seneca. *On the Shortness of Life*. Translated by C. D. N. Costa. New York: Penguin, 1997.

Shelley, Percy Bysshe. "Ode to the West Wind." https://www.poetryfoundation.org/poems/45134/ode-to-the-west-wind.

Shiel, William C., Jr. "Medical Definition of Hippocratic Oath." *Medicine Net*. https://www.medicinenet.com/script/main/art.asp?articlekey=20909.

Sinclair, David A., with Matthew D. LaPlante. *Life Span: Why We Age—and Why We Don't Have To*. New York: Atria, 2019.

Vanier, Jean. *The Scandal of Service: Jesus Washes Our Feet*. New York: Continuum, 1998.

Wallace, David Foster. "Interview." 2003. https://www.historyvshollywood.com/video/david-foster-wallace-interview.

"What is the definition of disability under the ADA?" *National Network ADA*. https://adata.org/faq/what-definition-disability-under-ada.

"World Report on Disability." *World Health Organization*. https://www.who.int/disabilities/world_report/2011/report/en/.

Yeats, William Butler. *The Collected Works of W. B. Yeats Volume 3: Autobiographies*. New York: Scribner, 2010.

Zec, Milica, dir. *Marina Abramovic on the Artist Is Present*. New York: Marina Abramovic Institute, 2010.

Made in United States
Orlando, FL
03 March 2023